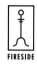

FIRESIDE

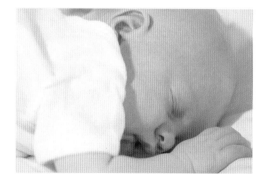

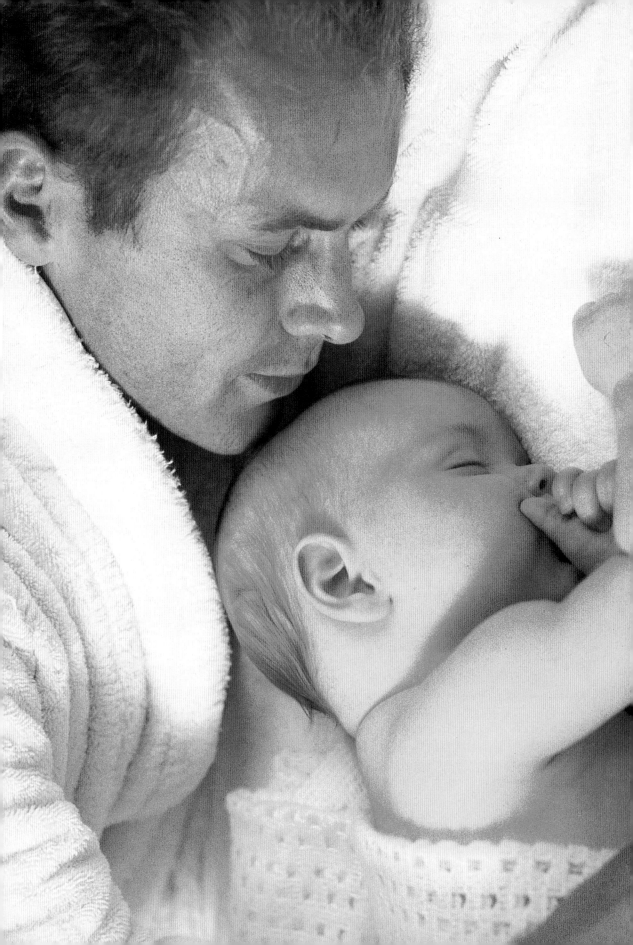

The

FertilityPlan

A Holistic Program *for* Conceiving

a Healthy Baby

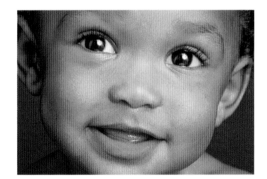

Helen Caton

with Damien Downing *and* Harold Buttram

A Fireside Book
Published by Simon and Schuster
New York   London   Sydney   Singapore

FIRESIDE
Rockefeller Center
1230 Avenue of the Americas
New York, NY 10020

To my daughter, Faith

FIRESIDE and colophon are registered trademarks
of Simon & Schuster, Inc.

Designed by Phil Gamble

Manufactured in Singapore by Kyodo

10 9 8 7 6 5 4 3 2 1

Note to Readers
This publication contains the opinions and ideas of its author.
It is intended to provide helpful and informative material on the
subjects addressed in the publication. It is sold with the
understanding that the author and publisher are not engaged in
rendering medical, health, psychological or any other kind of
personal professional services in the book. The reader should
consult his or her medical, health or other competent
professional before adopting any of the suggestions in this book
or drawing inferences from it.

The author and the publisher specifically disclaim all
responsibility for any liability, loss or risk, personal or otherwise,
which is incurred as a consequence, directly or indirectly, of the
use and application of any of the contents of this book.

Library of Congress Cataloging-in-Publication Data is available.

ISBN 0-684-86944-6

Contents

Introduction

A baby is a wondrous gift, a source of joy and amazement. The greatest concerns of prospective parents are for the health of the mother and future baby. The gift of life is so precious that we do all we can to give our children the best start. The good news is that you can improve your fertility, and enjoy a problem-free pregnancy and a thriving baby, simply by planning for a healthy conception.

In today's busy world, with its stresses and strains, low fertility is a problem for some couples. Many take some time to conceive. "Preconceptional care" is the new term for one of the oldest conventions in society. It means thinking about your future children and preparing for them, even before you conceive.

This book is based on a natural approach that is helpful for all couples, whether or not you have previous experience of subfertility or difficulties in pregnancy. Aimed at both men and women, it is based on gentle, natural methods that work for you both, giving you the best chance for a healthy conception, pregnancy, and childbirth.

You will see how a twin-track strategy based on boosting your fertility and a comprehensive program of preconceptional care can maximize your chances of conception. The benefits will be enjoyed by you all. Parents will experience greater vitality, improved relaxation, and more energy to cope with the challenges of a new baby. Your child will benefit from an easier birth, higher nutritional levels, and less likelihood of birth or developmental problems.

Clinical diagnosis and improved diet are crucial elements of this program. It is important that any nutritional deficiencies you may have are identified and corrected, and that any medical conditions are addressed before conception. Maturing sperm and fertilized eggs require high levels of nourishment long before we are aware of this need.

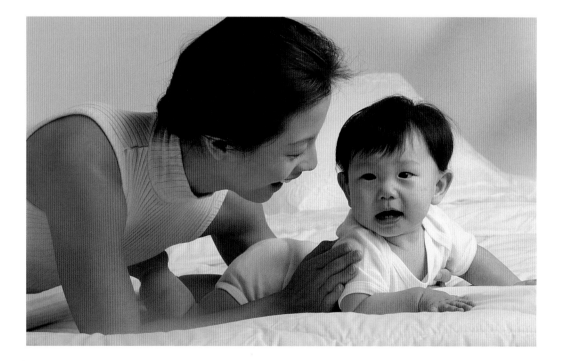

While nutritional supplements are necessary for some, a return to real food—preferably whole and organic—is recommended for all prospective parents. You will benefit from the higher nutritional levels, while avoiding artificial additives and other unwanted chemicals in processed foods. A diet high in vitamins and minerals also protects the body against the absorption of heavy metals, which can affect fertility.

The pressure of time passing is a worry for many couples and can create unnecessary levels of stress. To reduce or avoid this stress, you need a gentle pace: work toward a healthy conception when your bodies are ready. Rather than suggesting a "quick-fix" approach to conception, a more relaxed program is proposed here, building on your bodies' natural cycles of 28 days for women and about 90 for men. Once these cycles are established and a plan of action laid down for health, nutritional, and lifestyle improvements, the goal of a healthy conception is within sight.

If your clinician has indicated the need for assisted conception, there are still positive benefits from this approach to preconceptional care—it may even make assisted conception unnecessary. You can increase your likelihood of success by working through the various recommendations in this book. By raising your nutritional levels, relaxing, and introducing a healthier lifestyle, you will improve your chances. This program also offers support for those for whom assisted conception does turn out to be the best solution.

Complementary health care approaches are playing an increasingly important role in today's society. Ancient techniques are being rediscovered, and their benefits to overall health—and to fertility in particular—are being demonstrated. From aromatherapy massage to zone therapy, you can improve your general health, increase fertility levels, and successfully conceive, using holistic techniques.

This is a comprehensive care program that benefits from the active participation of both partners: man and woman. In addition to boosting your individual fertility levels, this partnership approach will strengthen and enhance your relationship. Your emotional needs are addressed, as well as your health and wellbeing. There are lifestyle changes to consider and opportunities to make improvements in your diet and exercise. By making these choices together, you will both feel supported and better able to focus on your goal of a healthier conception.

Preconceptional care can assist you in your future choice of birth control, too. By raising your fertility awareness, you can be liberated from over-reliance on chemical contraceptive techniques and their unwanted side effects. A greater understanding of the way your bodies work will bring you back in touch with your own fertility cycles and free you to make future choices based on less invasive methods of contraception.

Preconceptional care

Much of the research basis of this book was founded on the Foresight approach to preconceptional care. Foresight is a charity registered in Britain which has worked tirelessly to improve the wellbeing of couples affected by infertility. It also raises awareness of the environmental problems connected with fertility and offers natural solutions. Since the 1980s, Foresight has commissioned research into preconceptional care and reviewed the literature. Their approach is now supported by scientific evidence from around the world.

The science on which the Foresight approach is based is really common sense: diagnose deficiencies and improve the health

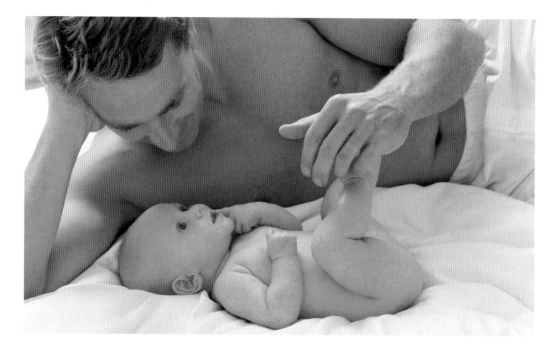

of both parents at the time when the male sperm and female egg are maturing (about 90 days before conception). The result is an improvement in fertility rates and a reduction in pregnancy—and birth—problems.

This would be an amazing claim, were it not borne out by research carried out at the University of Surrey, England. This tracked the progress of 367 couples who undertook the Foresight program between 1990 and 1992 and who were followed up in 1993.

Over a third of these couples had previously suffered from infertility—for up to ten years—or from pregnancy difficulties, such as miscarriage or premature birth. Tests showed that many of the male partners had reduced sperm quality. The follow-ups revealed a remarkable contrast: all babies were born healthy; they were well-developed at birth with a good birth weight and free from problems that might have required transfer to a special baby unit. Using the Foresight approach, 86 percent of couples with previous infertility problems achieved healthy pregnancies.

But this research does not show only the benefits to parents with a history of infertility. Couples without previous fertility problems can benefit from overall improved health, just as much as prospective parents in the older age group. Without resorting to chemical and hormonal stimulants or mechanical and often stressful medical treatments, couples can be confident of a good success rate and a high-quality pregnancy and birth.

About this book

This book takes you through the facts you need to improve your awareness about male and female fertility, to boost your fertility, and to integrate mental, physical, and spiritual considerations into your preparation.

Chapter 1 invites you to consider what it means to be ready for parenthood and looks at the emotional and practical considerations. Having taken a conscious decision to commit yourselves to a healthy conception, Chapter 2 shows how you can boost your health and fertility in five key steps. Chapter 3 is a practical introduction to male and female fertility awareness to help you to understand your bodies better.

You can further enhance your wellbeing by preparing holistically, selecting from the choice of complementary health care approaches described in Chapter 4. Chapter 5 brings all these elements together in a "countdown to conception" timetable that you can adapt to suit your particular circumstances. The first appendix looks at some current methods of assisted conception and explains how the recommendations in this book can work alongside an assisted conception program. A second appendix provides a fertility chart to copy and a sample of a lifestyle diary.

It must be stressed that this book takes its lead from the Foresight approach to preconceptional care, but is not intended as a substitute for professional medical advice. The information on complementary health care, for example, provides a taster for the different eastern and western approaches to health care, but it is recommended that you choose a complementary practitioner with experience of preconceptional care. Let your clinicians know what you're doing to improve your chances of conception.

Based on the principle that what is good for you is good for your future child, the approach contained in these pages is gentle yet effective. The aim of the countdown to conception is to help both of you achieve the best possible level of health in readiness for parenthood. By adapting your lifestyle, improving your diet and wellbeing, reducing hazards, and choosing flexible exercise routines, you can prepare for a successful and healthy conception.

The Foresight approach

Foresight clinicians are usually experienced practitioners, with a particular interest in the health and wellbeing of families. They may be doctors, nurses, midwives, or professional complementary practitioners, who have specialized in preconceptional care.

The Foresight approach is methodical and rigorous. Through changes in diet and lifestyle, it aims to promote healthy attitudes to future parenthood for the benefit of parents and children alike. Their research has been based on many studies of couples with a variety of reproductive problems, including those with a history of miscarriage and sudden infant death. The results continue to show an improved chance of conception, better health in pregnancy, and a host of bouncing babies for those who follow the regime.

Foresight has studied preconceptional care for many years and has identified a variety of factors that may cause problems in pregnancy, childbirth, and growth. The good news is that many of these factors can be avoided or successfully treated. The Foresight philosophy is to encourage overall good health and vitality, which in turn promotes a healthy conception.

If you were to attend a Foresight consultation, you would be asked to fill out out a questionnaire on your health and lifestyle and to take some diagnostic tests, including hair samples, for mineral analysis. A clinician would advise on nutrition and on vitamin and mineral supplements specially formulated for couples planning to conceive, and suggest simple lifestyle changes, such as filtering your drinking water, to improve your overall wellbeing.

Chapter one

Ready for parenthood?

Do you feel surrounded by friends and family members preparing for parenthood, by proud fathers-to-be discussing their role, and by future mothers comparing notes? For many couples, feeling left out is the greatest drive toward parenthood.

Parenthood involves positive decisions about how, where, and with whom you want to live—it isn't just about following your peer group. It raises spiritual as well as material matters. You may live in a society that offers you freedom of choice—when to start a family, when to wait—but with that comes a greater sense of responsibility to yourselves and your future children. You will want to give them the best possible start in life.

Many couples come under social pressure from parents, relatives, and friends to have children. Equally, there are many shared concerns—and a multitude of solutions. The issues covered in this chapter reflect a diversity of experiences from a variety of different people, from the standpoint that there is no one "right" answer for everyone. Planned parenthood is a personal choice for you as a couple.

The approach to preconceptional care outlined in this book has a high success rate in helping couples to conceive healthy children. For a few, though, parenthood is not appropriate or possible. Some couples are child-free by choice: it can be a positive option. By considering all the issues surrounding parenthood, you will have a greater control of your life choices. Of course, life has a funny knack of surprising us—sometimes delightfully, sometimes sadly. Be prepared to face what the future brings and allow yourself to enjoy life to the full.

Later sections of this book help you boost your fertility; this chapter looks at the parenting issues that may affect you. Use them as a starting point for building your confidence and discussing your concerns with your partner. It's only natural to be anxious about uncertainties, but don't let scare stories or self-doubt rob you of the joys of life. Your commitment is the key to maximizing your natural fertility. If you need more information about particular subjects, use the reference section at the end of the book for sources and helpful organizations.

Deciding whether or not to start a family is a matter for you and your partner. Discussing parenting issues with your friends and family can also be helpful, but don't let yourselves feel pressurized.

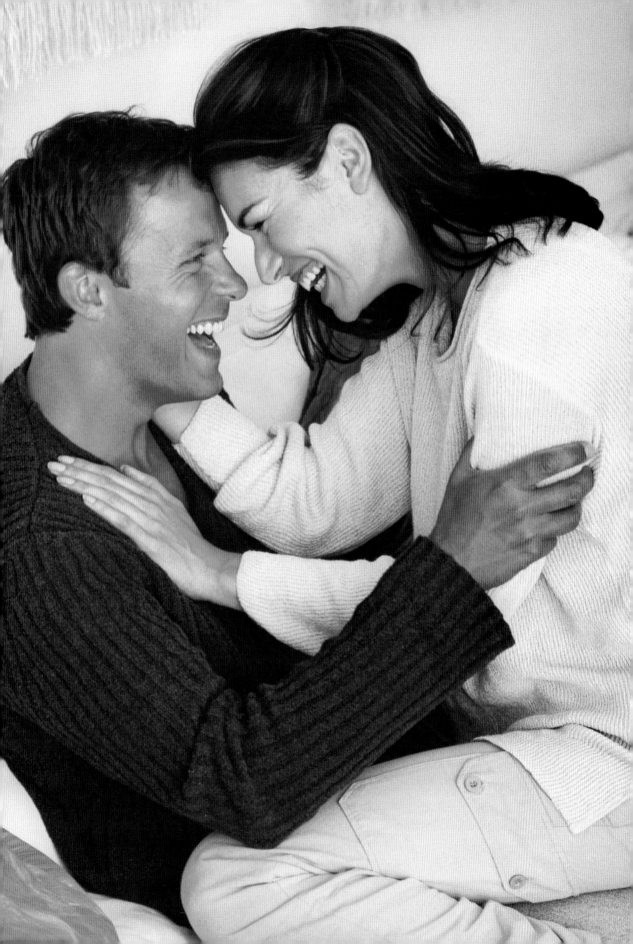

Taking time out to talk

Remember why you first found each other so attractive, why you wanted to be together? Good communication is often the key to good partnerships, and successful relationships are founded on the ability to share thoughts and freely exchange views. People whom we can trust with our emotions and innermost fears are the most special to us—our "best friends."

After a while, it is easy to forget these fundamental points and stop making time to talk. If you want to raise the subject of having a baby with your partner, now is the moment to bring good communications back into your relationship. If you have been trying to conceive a child for some time, there may be some sensitive and personal issues you still need to talk over. Discuss ways of improving your preconceptional care, then take the practical steps together.

It is vital to find ways of talking about your relationship that take both of your points of view into account. It is well known that men and women vary in the way they use language. Men are typically trained to use a logical approach, which seems (to some women) to take subjects literally, rather than using them as ways to express and explore issues. Women, on the other hand, are often accused of making generalizations, or of being over-dramatic and not dealing with "the facts."

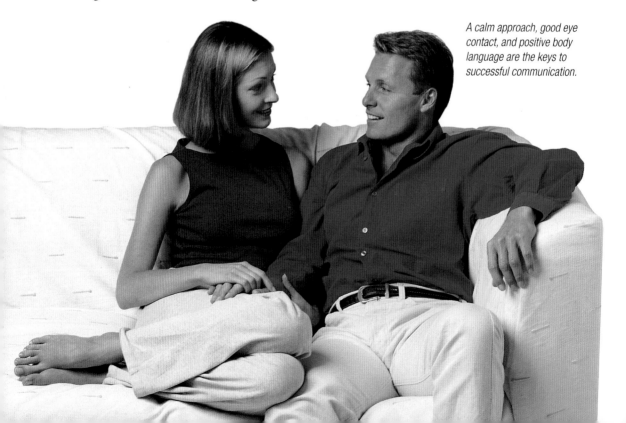

A calm approach, good eye contact, and positive body language are the keys to successful communication.

Fears can be overcome only by focusing on the moment, not by dwelling on what was, or what might be. Women may worry that time is running out for them; men may fear having a sperm test, or finding out the results. Partnerships are about trust: there is no point in expressing false confidence or trying to cover up your nervousness about a difficult topic—particularly one that affects both you and future generations.

Prepare to talk by relaxing your mind and calming your emotions. In this way you will make yourself clear, even if you need to discuss a subject about which you are uncertain. Acknowledge the actions you would like, or expect, each other to take, whether it is booking an appointment with the fertility clinic or simply arranging to attend a yoga class together.

Your body language will have as much impact as your words. Eye contact, tone of voice, and touch are just as important as what you say. If you feel right about talking, it will be expressed in your voice, reflected in your eyes, and felt in the way you touch each other.

Above all, be ready at all times to express your love and affection for each other: don't take your partner for granted. Whatever decisions you make, make them together, on the basis of mutual affection and respect.

The right time...the right place

Find time to have unhurried discussions when you are both relaxed and ready to open up with each other—over a lazy Sunday brunch, for example. If you are rushed or under stress, you may feel that there is never a "right" moment. Late-night discussions, or moments snatched before an important business meeting, can be stressful and often inappropriate.

Avoid talking over important or complex subjects in the car—you can't look into each other's eyes and you won't be able to give the topic the concentration it deserves.

Making time means finding opportunities to relax and unwind—often after a busy day—when you can let the pressures of work, friends, and family drop away. If necessary, book some free hours together into your diaries. Switch on the answering machine and enjoy a delicious meal—set up a calm atmosphere in which you can really talk.

One way of dealing with sensitive subjects, such as sexual issues, is to initiate a lighthearted discussion, which can deal gently with tender problems. Broaching the subject in a unexpected or "neutral" situation, away from the bedroom, can help lighten the atmosphere. Express what you find good in each other. Use positive language, humor, and touch to emphasize how important your relationship is to you.

Dealing with your emotions

It is well recognized that women's fluctuating hormonal cycles affect their emotional state. What is less accepted is that real concerns often lie behind the expression of emotions. Emotional outbursts may be caused by the bottling up of anxiety and the failure to deal with issues as they arise. Distress may be unpredictable or unexpected, but the concerns that are being expressed are always valid.

It is also important to remember that men experience emotions, too. In western society the ability of men to express their innermost feelings varies, ranging from Latin cultures—where physical touch between men, a greater openness, and expression of feeling is commonplace—to northern Europe, where society is more restrained, as expressed in the stereotype of the Englishman and his "stiff upper lip."

Being clear about what you want to say

Clarity of thought will lead to clarity of expression. Take your time and, if necessary, plan in advance what you want to say and what you are trying to achieve. Some conversations have an end point—an objective—while others may be more like a brainstorming session. The important thing is to avoid talking around and around a subject, without coming to a conclusion.

If you're feeling "stuck" and finding it difficult even to articulate your fears or concerns, think about booking a relaxation session. This might be with an aromatherapist using essential oils, or even in a floatation tank, where many poets and songwriters formulate their ideas. See Chapter 4 for more ideas.

When you are ready to talk, focus on the subject that is your greatest priority. Although you may wish to tackle the whole subject of preconceptional care, pregnancy, and childbirth, it may not be possible to do so in the time you have available. You can still discuss individual topics in a holistic fashion, but it's better to do so in manageable "bites."

It's important to be direct when communicating, using humor or affection to reassure your partner. Be clear and specific in expressing what you want and use the "I feel" phrase to explain your feelings. Avoid speaking for your partner; instead invite him or her to state their own feelings and desires. At the end of your discussion, you should both feel you have spent some time talking, some time listening, and that you have both participated in the decisions you have reached.

Make sure you are in agreement about principles before you move on to actions. Also, make sure that you both understand the reasons why you need to take action. Expecting your partner to attend a clinic for tests before you have both agreed to the idea of conception, or discussed the benefits of tests, may come as a serious shock.

One or the other of you may want to delay making a particular decision until you have more facts. This may necessitate making a phone call, getting a book out of the library, or finding out some medical background from a family member. Even if you've got some difficult news to report, don't put off sharing it. The sooner you know the facts, the sooner you can get on with finding a way to deal with them—together.

Steps to good communications

Saying what you mean can be difficult when the subject is so personal. Brush up on your communication skills with these tips:

Do:

- Be clear about your topic and stick to the subject.
- Make time to communicate in an open and relaxed atmosphere.
- Take responsibility for how you feel and use phrases that reflect this, such as "I feel that…"
- Suggest a range of solutions to problems—there is always an alternative.
- Plan actions in manageable steps.

Don't:

- Transfer your feelings to your partner with such expressions as "you make me feel…."
- Talk about complex, sensitive subjects while driving.
- Take, or allocate, blame—think about solutions.
- Delay telling difficult news or delay important decisions simply for fear of hurting your partner's feelings.
- Use negative language, such as "you don't…," "you never…," "we can't…." Remain constructive.

Have a "brainstorming" session

Brainstorming allows you to explore ideas, as they arise and
without restraint. Try it when you are both feeling relaxed
and in the mood to be expansive and talkative. Pick a subject—
whether it's your lifestyle or what it means to be a parent—
and explore your concerns together.

Let all your ideas and concerns come up—without pre-
judging them. Write them down just as they arise. Agree to
remain uncritical until you have exhausted all your ideas. Then
take a good look. Are there particular topics coming up again
and again? Are there any major concerns that impact on your
place of work, or your home? Even the silliest-sounding phrase
may have the germ of a good idea in it.

What are your agreed outcomes? It might be to visit your
medical adviser, spend more time together, or find a dance class;
it may be agreeing to talk over your concerns about parenthood
with family or friends. In reality, these are just steps along the
way, rather than conclusions, but taking the first steps together
will give you both confidence—whatever you plan to do.

Typical discussion topics

Ray and Sandy are in their late thirties, and typical of many
parents who have one child but then experience complications.
"We are very happy together, but we wanted to make the
relationship more 'complete' by having a baby. I was very
fortunate to succeed after a year of trying, and Susie, our four
year old, is such a joy to be with—naturally we wanted to try
again. When I miscarried a year later, I was devastated; the
physical and emotional trauma was almost overwhelming.
Now I look back and count my blessings: I have a loving,
caring husband and a happy, healthy child."

It's likely that Sandy's nutritional levels were low when she
conceived the second time; she had a young baby to look after
and was constantly exhausted. After the miscarriage, Sandy's
periods stopped altogether, and it took a regime of herbal
medicine to restore her cycle.

Sandy has talked the situation through with Ray, and they
have looked into the choice of natural preconceptional care
approaches. "If I conceive again in the coming year, it will be
as a result of my herbal treatments, shiatsu, and our more
relaxed lifestyle combined. We've also studied fertility awareness,
and we've got a good routine going charting my cycle."

While doing all they can to boost their fertility levels, Ray
and Sandy have also considered the possibility of not conceiving:

"If I don't succeed, I'm not going to keep on and on. We'll explain the situation to Susie and get on with our lives."

Your situation may be made up of a different set of issues, such as parental concerns, financial constraints, or simply the desire to be as healthy as possible when you conceive. Here are some typical concerns that parents-to-be raise in discussion:

Why do we want to conceive?

We want to express our love for each other and complete our relationship. By having a child you will "add" to the relationship in a number of ways, dividing your time, affection, and attention between two or more people, instead of just one. Remember that you are already complete individuals. As a couple you have a whole relationship; having a child will not make you more so. Feel your existing completeness first and then decide whether to make room for a new life in your relationship.

Our parents would really like for us to make them grandparents. For some couples this is a pressure, whether expressed or unspoken. Your parents may want to be reassured that there is still a role for them within the family circle now that their task of bringing you up is over. They may be looking forward to the unconditional love that is somehow easier to give to grandchildren than children. Or they may just want to let you know that they will be there for you if and when you do decide to become parents. Let them express their desires and acknowledge their feelings, but don't allow yourselves to be unduly pressured by their expectations.

We want someone to love and to love us. Love is a personal, individual, inner experience. It is a state of being, the source of which is within ourselves—not "out there" somewhere. Our partners, parents, and friends reflect that experience, and we can share our affection, but it's important to be in touch with the source of love within you.

Another human being cannot "give" you love; you have to feel it first inside yourself and then express it. Babies are particularly demanding: they will give you sleepless nights and interrupted meals, draining your mental and physical resources. Even so, when you bond with your baby in the midst of it all, you will experience a deep connection. The reason we find it so easy to adore babies is that the interaction is so straightforward, rewarding, and totally unconditional. Babies exude love—it's their nature—and we respond to that.

I think it will improve our relationship. Sadly, many partners see a valued relationship foundering and decide that having a child will save it. This is often far from the case. If you are feeling unsteady, you can be sure your partner feels it, too. Talk about your relationship and how much it means to you. Invest in it and achieve positive stability first. Having a child simply in the hope that he or she will shore up a difficult relationship is just not realistic. An innocent, vulnerable child can't sort out your problems—you need adult, professional help. It can be a positive decision, not a failure, to delay having a child until you are both ready to take this major step.

Are we ready to become parents?

Are we old enough? Biologically, young people can conceive in their teens, but it is accepted that they are often too immature to appreciate fully the responsibilities of parenthood.

Puberty is related to a growth spurt, triggered by a complex series of factors related to weight. Young men need to reach a "critical metabolic mass" related to a body weight of at least 120 pounds. This figure may be higher, depending on factors such as the young man's skeletal frame, body fat, and lean body weight. For women, the figure is at least 100 pounds and is constant, not related to age. Good nutrition is the key to physical maturity, although social conditions and health care are also important factors.

Physiologically, the best time for conception is when the prospective parents are at least in their mid-twenties. For the mother-to-be, this is when her system is physically mature enough to cope with the stresses and strains of childbirth and the endurance test of bringing up a child. Men typically progress through adolescence at a different rate and may not be fully physically matured until their mid-twenties.

Are we emotionally mature enough to have a child? Gauging emotional maturity is more complex than estimating physical development. Emotions are often presented as fickle feelings, at odds with rational intelligence. In reality they are triggered by a combination of hormones and neural responses, and they fluctuate with hormonal cycles and nutritional levels in both men and women. Maturity is not necessarily about controlling emotions; instead, it is about taking them into account when reaching decisions.

If you feel that you communicate well as a couple and are ready to make responsible choices together, based on thoughtful, shared decisions and backed up with practical actions, then you are probably mature enough to become parents.

Are we leaving it too late?

This case study is an example of a happy ending after many years of struggle. Michael and Annette Banyard gave up trying to have children after 23 years of marriage and were totally surprised when Annette's "stomach pains" heralded the arrival of Jason, a healthy baby weighing six pounds! After two miscarriages, Annette had tried fertility treatment for eight years without success, "…we lost hope and gave up and that seemed to be the end of it."

Michael feels that a change of lifestyle may have been an important factor: "I think living on a canal boat has done us good. We're out in the countryside, the air is clean, and there's no stress." Doctors are amazed—and delighted—by Michael and Annette's achievement: "It is a remarkable story," said consultant obstetrician and gynecologist Martin Powell of the Queen's Medical Centre, Nottingham, England. "To become

Probably the best time to start a family is when your relationship has had time to mature—typically, after three years of a stable, committed partnership.

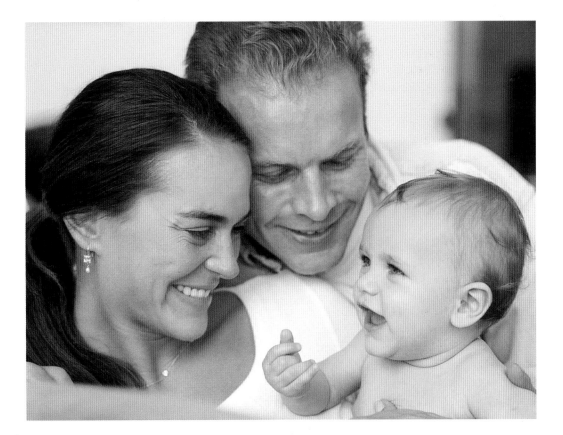

pregnant at this point is a minor miracle. What is even more fantastic is that Jason is a healthy child."

I'm coming up to 40. Is it too late to think about bearing my first child? Female fertility peaks in the mid-twenties, and statistically the older the woman, the longer it will take her to conceive. Many women are delaying the decision to start a family, which does create some uncertainty about fertility. However, there are plenty of examples of women bearing their first healthy child at 40, with no problems at all. Crucial factors are the quality of the maturing egg and getting enough nourishment to sustain the moment of conception and the all-important early days of the fetus.

Your family medical history, particularly on the female side, will play an important part in your decision. It is also vital that you take the advice of your clinician, since some birth problems are linked to age as much as to your wellbeing. Think about the tests you may undergo to check for fetal abnormalities and the consequences of a positive result. Be clear in your own mind, and discuss everything with your medical adviser and partner first, before deciding what to do.

I've heard that sperm quality declines as a man gets older. Is this true?
It's true that fertility declines with age in men, although at a slower rate than for women. However, in the same way that women rely on nutritional input to produce high-quality eggs, the quality of male sperm is also linked to good nutrition. Concerns have been expressed that men over 50 may produce sperm that passes on defective DNA, but tests are now commonly available and can help you come to a decision.

Does the potential age gap between us and our child matter?
In addition to the ability to father or bear a child, you will need the strength to nurture it. The first few months of a child's life are like a prolonged endurance test for parents. Just establishing a routine is hard enough, and then you will need still more energy to play with your child. Later, when your child goes to school, you will be invited to participate in parent-teacher and other social activities, and it is your drive and commitment that will count, not necessarily your age. If you do decide to try to conceive, find ways of keeping yourselves in tiptop condition. Enhance your natural vitality and aim to break down those conventional age barriers.

Freedom and responsibility

Could we cope with the responsibility? The responsibility for the care of a child is absolute and could be summed up as fulfilling your baby's needs, physically and emotionally, for 24 hours every day. But this is a shared task. Not only parents but also friends and neighbors typically want to take part—let them! Knowing when to give your all is as important as knowing when to let others take some responsibility. Over time, you will teach your children how to be self-reliant and to do everything for themselves. Then comes the hardest task of all: letting go.

Will we lose our freedom? The demands of parenthood will shift your focus from many of the social pleasures enjoyed when you were single, toward more home-centered activities. But this does not mean that you will never enjoy a late-night party, rock concert, or spectacular firework display again! Planning is the key, and once you develop a network of trusted sitters, you can select those social activities that mean most to you.

Will a child threaten the stability of our relationship? Consider the influences of other people on your lives. Do you discuss visiting your parents or parents-in-law together, or having them to stay? Do you talk about the impact of different friends and family members on your way of life? A child can sometimes be like an uninvited guest, turning up at the most inconvenient moment; for others, it is like a longed-for gift that fulfills your greatest expectations. Of course, a baby will upset all the routines you have spent years nurturing—but isn't that part of the fun? Learning to balance your own needs—and those of your partner—with the demands of your baby is a process that takes time and commitment. Sometimes you will get the balance wrong and one of you will feel a little left out. In a mature, considerate relationship, you can adapt, adjust, and make the space necessary to make sure you are all getting the affection and attention you need.

What about our older children?

Our first child is eight now. What about the age gap between the children? Views about age gaps are conditioned by your experience of what is "normal." It is essential that all the children in a family feel they are loved, and this means repeated reassurance. Treating children as individuals means allowing them to develop relationships with their own peer groups—at all ages. For example, taking a child's best friend along on a family outing will help him or her develop an independent identity and provide a secure social context. Children need to develop their own relationship with a younger sibling at their own pace. It is important not to pressure them with your expectations. Some children will feel very close to their younger siblings; others will be at a stage when friends or other interests are more important.

What if the older children develop "sibling rivalry"? Feelings of jealousy toward the new baby are more apparent during the first seven years of life, but older children may still experience them. You can prepare yourselves for any jealousy by planning your strategy and asking friends and family what worked for them. Children under five will not be able to articulate their feelings: they may manifest their fears by becoming clinging or possessive, or they may revert to "baby talk" or babyish behavior. Try using play to encourage younger children to act out their feelings. Once they feel comfortable and secure again, they will, typically, leave these habits behind.

Older children may show an outward acceptance of change but harbor inner resentments. You can encourage them to draw

The arrival of a new baby can be a shock for older children, however well they have been prepared. They will need reassurance that you still have plenty of time and love for them.

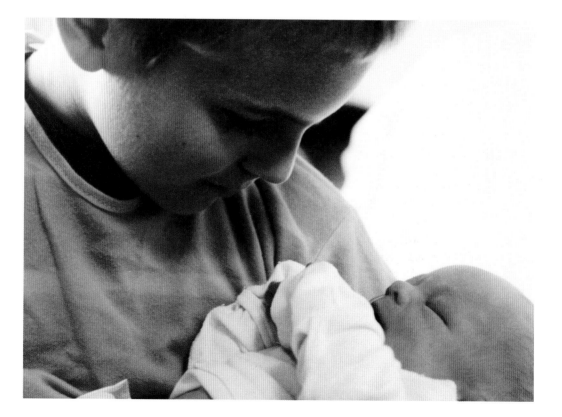

pictures or act out their feelings with dolls. Whatever their age, talk through your plans with your older children, in a language they can relate to. Give them time to think about what you've said and a chance to express their hopes and fears about any forthcoming changes. Reassure them in ways that are truthful and meaningful. Be specific about details in reply to questions such as "where will the new baby sleep?" Share with them the practicalities that you will have to consider.

This is a second marriage for both of us. We would like another child, but want our existing children to feel included. How can we help them? Today, extended families are more often created through divorce than the death of a parent. Since this means that adults and children alike have suffered some pain in the transition, and there is a surviving parent, sensitivity is crucial. Love is the essential starting point, and constant reassurance that the children are in no way to blame for the breakdown of the earlier relationship is necessary.

Children hate insecurity: make sure they know that they are all loved and wanted, and that future babies will not exclude them. Let your actions match your words: spending time with your children individually and planning shared activities together will show them that you mean what you say.

Practical considerations

Can we afford a child? Children consume their parents' income at an alarming rate! You may find that items previously taken for granted become occasional luxuries. What happens is a process of "diversion," whereby your financial resources are being diverted into your future child. This happens when you save for a new home, for example, possibly long before you conceive. When your baby is expected, you may spend time and effort preparing the nursery. The main reason that parents are happy for this to happen is that it feels more like "investment" than "expenditure," where the returns come in the form of loving family relationships.

Think about the role the prospective grandparents may wish to play. Perhaps they can help out with major items as a way of participating in your future child's wellbeing? If they are not so well off, they may want to offer more practical support.

If you have serious money problems, such as financial over-commitments or the prospect of losing your job, explore what steps you can take to restore stability before you start a family. You might decide to cut out some expenditure or reduce your credit-card debts. Losing your job might turn out to be a timely opportunity to consider childcare options if you are both agreed about how you will manage your future finances.

Will we have to move house? The availability of suitable accommodation, closely linked to career opportunities and access to facilities such as healthcare and education, is often a worry for parents-to-be. It's important to remember that social networks, such as family and friends, are just as important as practical matters in this context. Moving to a "better" neighborhood may leave you feeling isolated in the future if your close friends or family are at a distance. Do your best to strike a balance between the selection of local facilities and resources, and your overall quality of life.

What childcare support do we need? Support networks are vital to your own wellbeing and the development of your future children. You will need to come to a decision between the two of you as to who might stay at home. When looking for further support, your family and friends will probably be your first point of contact. Check local information sources for registered daycare facilities. Your employers may provide a work place

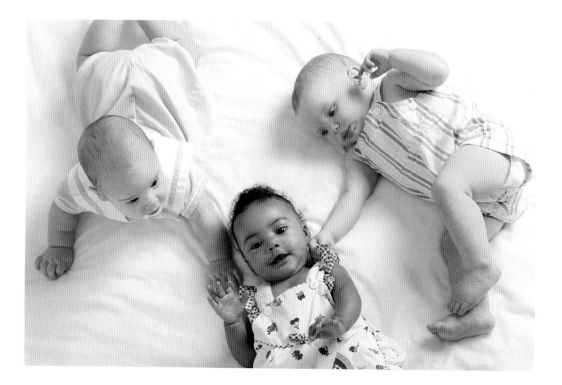

nursery or contribute in some way to childcare costs. If you want to employ a nanny, whether living in or out, you will need to find out about tax and social security contributions. Your local library will be a good source of information.

Whichever option you choose, be clear about your carer's role and the tasks you expect to be undertaken. If you are away all day, your children will form emotional attachments to those who are more central to their daily activities. Be prepared to balance your working day by spending quality time with your children in activities that are meaningful to them, whether routine or special treats, work or play.

What about our careers?

Should I put my career "on hold"? Think about the practical and financial considerations, as well as the intellectual stimulation your job offers. Look at your partner's job as well and compare the two. Increasingly, many men, as well as women, put their career on hold in order to become parents. Now that many women are in senior positions of responsibility, it is not always the automatic choice for the mother to stay at home once the baby is born.

With the current pace of change, a prolonged period away from the workplace will undoubtedly have an impact. Before you make your decision, check what your future position would be and whether any other options are available. You may find that you could work parttime, which would allow you to combine a satisfying career with the pleasures of parenthood. You may have the same general rights as a fulltime employee, such as joining an occupational pension plan and employment protection, but it is important to check your state's latest laws, since these can change.

You may also consider reducing your hours during your countdown to conception, in order to improve your chances. This is particularly relevant if your medical history suggests that you need to boost your fertility.

There are two typical options for parttime work: reducing your hours or organizing a job-share. There are important benefits in returning parttime, both for employer and employee: organizations retain good-quality, trained staff; you are likely to be more effective and stimulated by the work environment; and you can help cover busy periods.

Some points to consider before you decide: sometimes part-time workers do more hours than they are paid for—time spent handing over work, for example; promotion prospects may be reduced, and there may be less time or fewer resources for training you. Your salary level may affect your social security record, and you may have to work longer hours than before to achieve overtime rates of pay.

Once you have considered these options, get the support of your colleagues and your supervisor or manager, as well as your union, if you belong to one. They will have experience of similar situations and can advise you further, as well as helping you negotiate with your employer.

Check how much notification you must give your employer, and be sure to get into the habit of putting things in writing. It may seem a long way off, but if you do not reply to written requests for notification, you may lose your right to return to work after the birth of your baby.

Legal rights to parental leave

What are our maternity leave rights? It may be that your state has "statutory maternity rights," which may be available to all working mothers-to-be, regardless of their length of service at work. These rights should allow you time off and the right to return to your employment once the baby is born. Maternity rights vary from place to place and you should check the rules that apply locally. Your library will probably have this information. Also check your entitlement to other benefits:

- Maternity benefits: these provide a small regular sum for a period up to and beyond childbirth. They are typically available for those who have been with an employer for a specified minimum length of time.
- Improved contracts of employment: employers can negotiate improvements, but they cannot take statutory rights away.
- Protection from dismissal: it can be unlawful to dismiss an employee on the grounds of pregnancy or recent childbirth, or if you are ill following statutory maternity leave.

The main rights you can expect—although they will vary from place to place—are:

- Paid time off for prenatal care, which may include attendance at medical examinations, appointments with your clinician, and relaxation classes.
- Protection against unfair dismissal or loss of job, purely on maternity-related grounds.
- "Maternity leave," which is usually for those with less than two years' continuous employment, and "maternity absence," for employees with two years' continuous employment who are entitled to extended leave of absence.

■ Maternity benefits, which are dependent upon length
  of service and contributions paid.

Do fathers have any paternity leave rights? There is increasing
support for equal rights of leave for both future parents. These
are known as "parental leave" rights, and this is a new area of
legislation in many countries, notably member states of the
European Union. If there is no law where you live, there are
still ways in which you can arrange time off with your employer.
You could negotiate, perhaps with the help of a trade union,
anything from a few days of unpaid vacation through to full
transfer of maternity rights, if the father is to be the main carer
for your future child. Your contract of employment may allow
you to take a period of special or compassionate leave (with or
without pay), which you might be able to use to take time off
at the time of the birth.

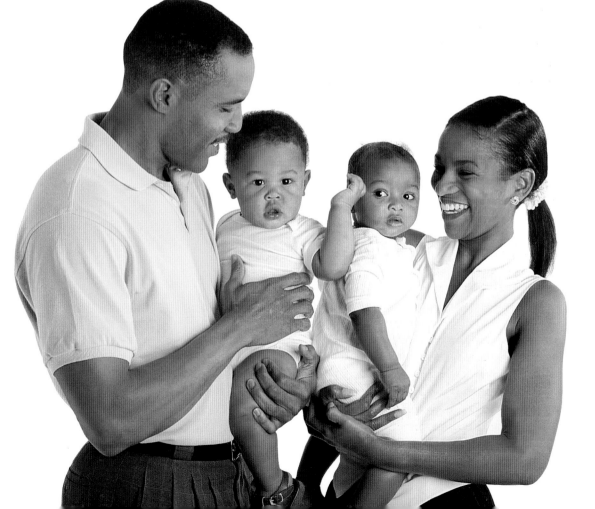

If you don't have any contractual rights to additional time off and can't manage to come to an agreement with your employer, see if you can arrange to have your annual vacation around the forthcoming event.

What do we do if we're told we're "infertile?" This is an unspoken fear of many couples wishing to become parents. Some men are reluctant even to undergo tests because of the potentially enormous blow to their self-esteem if they are told they have a low or zero sperm count. For women, it is a concern that is always at the back of their minds.

First of all, remember that one in six couples seeks help with fertility. It is not an uncommon concern. Of these, many go on to conceive naturally, with a little bit of practical advice or information on how our bodies work. Dr. Damien Downing, who has a practice in London, sees many couples in this situation. He says, "Typically, the couples I see have been told that the problem resides in one or the other partner. When we investigate, we find that in around two-thirds of all such cases neither partner is infertile, but both are 'subfertile' (see pages 82–85), which is much more treatable." The advice to "go away and keep trying" is a common response, and sometimes that's all you will need. But if that doesn't work, the information in this book may help you pinpoint a particular problem, such as an irregular ovulation cycle or the need to boost your sperm count.

Coming off the pill or IUD is another typical problem. You expect conception to be instantaneous, but of course your body is adjusting to its normal hormonal or mineral levels. Remember that cells take at least a month to absorb fully any vitamin and mineral supplements, and that sperm has a cycle of about 90 days. Regular dietary and supplement routines are vital.

But if, over time, your friends become pregnant and another month goes by without your conceiving, don't suppress your disappointment. Find someone you can really talk to, perhaps an understanding friend or a professional counselor.

The medical profession will never say "never," but neither can they give you a cast-iron guarantee of success. They will offer you all the tests and treatments within their power, and as long as you understand the treatment process, you will undoubtedly find the determination to go through with it. Hospital appointments, treatment regimes, trials, and disappointments are part of a stressful cycle. You can break this cycle through relaxation techniques and complementary treatments. Take charge of your choices and opt to enjoy your life—right now.

Of course, if at any time you decide that enough is enough and you want to stop trying to conceive—have the courage of your convictions. Know what is right for both of you, even if that means taking some difficult decisions and telling your parents or friends about your choice. You already have a precious life—your own. You can use it to benefit from the pleasure of other people's children or to help humanity in your own special way. Having a child is not the only way to bring love and joy into your life.

Finally, always leave some room in your life for a miracle… whether it is the joy of childbirth or the simple pleasures of living each day to the full. Keep space free for surprises, and watch the magic unfold.

A success story

This is a true story, told to me by a mother who wanted other couples to know that, even in the face of many difficulties, it is possible to conceive and have a normal delivery. Here is her story in Franses' own words.

"Grayham and I tried for a year before our first conception, but we were unable to keep the pregnancy. I cried for more than two weeks after my first miscarriage and felt a failure. After several more miscarriages, a referral to a fertility specialist (who advised us that my husband had a lower-than-average sperm count) and visits to a counselor, I felt that we had to do something to help ourselves. We had read about the benefits of vitamins and minerals, but we wanted a regime and expert support from someone who really knew about these things, so we made an appointment to see a clinician who was a specialist in preconceptional care.

I became pregnant again before the appointment, so the treatment was aimed at helping me keep the pregnancy. Tests showed that we were deficient in a lot of vitamins and minerals, particularly B12 and calcium, and we were advised about what to take. The dietary approach seemed natural. We already filtered our water, and we began to cut out foods with unwanted additives. We changed our bread and switched to decaffeinated tea. The hospital recommended an aspirin daily as they felt it would benefit my situation. It's hard to describe how I felt. We became very cautious during the pregnancy, taking our doctor's advice to 'take each day as it comes.' I was afraid to buy anything for the baby. I was continually sick for 13 weeks, but I was happy to be sick because at least I was still pregnant!

The outcome? We now have a beautiful baby boy, Christian, who was born at 40 weeks. He is like a miracle for us—what more can I say?

The future? We're still taking the vitamins and following our changed diet and recommended 'maintenance program.' We hope that one day we might give Christian a brother or sister. I now feel able to be a practical help to my family and friends in a similar position."

Franses' story is very special, but not unique. I hear many wonderful stories of couples conceiving apparently "against the odds." Remember, there are no guarantees of success or of a problem-free pregnancy, but the advice in this book can help you maximize your chances.

What about our medical history?

There are specific medical issues to take into consideration when planning a pregnancy, as Chapters 2 and 3 point out, and some of these are listed below. The approach to preconceptional care outlined in this book will help all couples improve their general health, but you may have an existing condition that appears to stack the odds against you.

- Infertility is seldom an inevitable consequence of illness or major medical treatments, but it is important to have a thorough medical checkup. Be prepared for a full battery of tests for preexisting infections and other conditions. Knowing your family history will be very useful at this point, and if you can pinpoint the dates of your own medical history, your doctor will be in a better position to diagnose and treat underlying conditions that may affect your fertility.
- Infections, sometimes referred to as "inflammatory diseases," may be without symptoms. Chlamydia and candidiasis can affect fertility in men and women, and your doctor may treat you both to make sure any infection is eradicated. Common infections like these can deplete your immune system, and fertility is often the first thing to be affected.
- For women, a previous ectopic pregnancy (possibly linked to previous use of an IUD) may seem like an insurmountable hurdle to conception. Other gynecological problems, such as previous pelvic inflammatory disease or endometriosis, may leave a woman with scarred or infected tubes.
- Men may be rendered infertile by certain surgical and cancer treatment techniques, as well as by catching childhood diseases, such as mumps, in later life. In the case of cancer treatments, with careful planning, healthy sperm can be developed and "banked" by prospective fathers as an insurance against possible future infertility.

Before you begin your countdown, it is important to address these issues sensitively. Men may feel that their virility is threatened by the idea of having tests. Women with previous abortions or miscarriages may feel guilty. There may be something in your past that your partner doesn't know about and that may affect your ability to conceive. You may have an hereditary condition which you don't even know about yet.

Most adults have been through life experiences that they would prefer not to think about. By coming to terms with your medical history, you can improve your chances of a healthy conception. You can't change the past, but this is your opportunity to change the future—for yourselves, for each other and for your future children.

Some conditions that may affect fertility

Jackie suffers from MS and had her first attack when her first baby was less than a year old. She is now expecting her second child. Like many MS sufferers, she enjoys a close relationship with others in her situation and downloads a lot of information from the Internet, including information on complementary therapies. She explains, "Most information is very balanced— not trying to sway your decision either way. I read up a lot on my condition once I'd been diagnosed, and I respect the views of others. I feel very positive about my decision to have another baby. I'm currently six months pregnant, and thanks to a lot of support from my husband and family, I'm doing well!"

Jackie is also very positive about the power of counseling, particularly from trained volunteers. "They understand our situation and speak to couples like us every week. We just need advice on coping strategies or ways of handling particular symptoms; it helps us get on with living a normal life."

Many people suffering from medical conditions share Jackie's

You may already have discussed your concerns with your clinician. Some prospective parents, on the other hand, may not be aware of preexisting conditions, and this is why thorough tests are important.

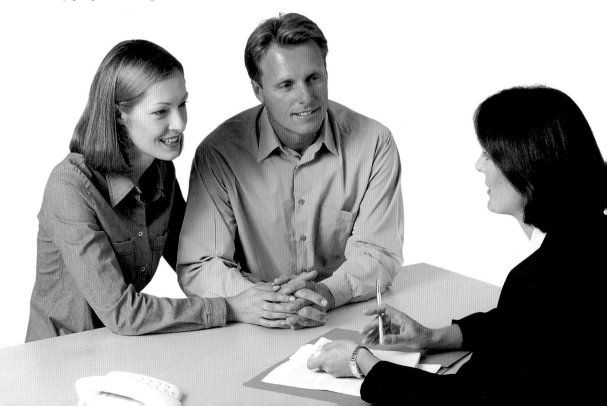

pragmatic approach and won't let their illness detract from life's pleasures. Stress can make symptoms worse. Self-help strategies that deal with practical situations will reduce your anxiety and restore confidence, particularly if you know they have worked for other people with your condition.

If you have any kind of diagnosed condition, making sure you have a balanced diet is particularly important and will help your overall health as well as your fertility. Complementary treatments (see Chapter 4) can help stabilize your condition and improve some symptoms, particularly if you are suffering from sexual problems as a side-effect. Complementary treatments may also help you to reduce your medication levels, but they should always be carried out in consultation with your doctor.

Multiple Sclerosis (MS)

MS sufferers are sometimes faced with sexual function problems, associated with neurological and emotional causes. Fatigue is also a common problem, which may affect sexual drive, and some people may lack sensation. Sexual activity does not make MS worse, but overtiredness may exacerbate some symptoms. These problems may lead to men being unable to maintain an erection and may cause women to feel stressed or inadequate, but underlying fertility is not usually affected.

To combat this, consider alternative, more restful, lovemaking positions. Reassure each other, remembering that most adults will feel less inclined toward sex when they are feeling stressed. Make sure the partner with MS has regular rests and a good balanced diet. Use complementary therapies to relax you and reduce your symptoms—both of you will benefit. Pace your daily activities, and if you decide to go ahead and conceive, seek assistance from your friends, family, and support services.

Epilepsy

Fertility levels in people suffering from epilepsy are not necessarily affected, but there are problems associated with the anticonvulsant drugs typically prescribed to patients. There are known links between prescribed drugs for epilepsy and fetal abnormalities. The risks can be reduced by minimizing prescription levels as early as possible. You should also make sure your nutrition is good at the time when you are planning to conceive. Optimum vitamin and mineral levels have a dual purpose: they will help reduce the number of epileptic episodes and make sure the developing egg has maximum nutritional supplies at the critical early stages.

There is also an interaction between the drugs used to treat epilepsy and the contraceptive pill, which leads to a more rapid breakdown of estrogen. This means that women suffering from epilepsy are typically prescribed higher doses of medication, which may have a knock-on effect on the time it takes to conceive. The problem can be countered by improving your nutritional levels when you are planning for conception, the avoidance of the birth-control pill, and the use of alternative birth-control methods until you are ready to conceive.

Kidney disease

A variety of conditions fall under the general heading of "kidney disease", some of which may affect the ability to have children. Pregnancy also puts additional pressure on the kidneys, so may worsen their function temporarily. A low-sodium diet may be necessary. Ask your specialist for guidance.

The most common problem is that of regulating blood pressure, which can benefit from self-help through relaxation techniques, as well as medical support. Some prescribed drugs may cause fetal abnormalities, and their use should be discussed with your clinician. In other cases, pregnancy may exacerbate symptoms, and before you proceed, you should consider carefully the advice you receive.

Improved clinical care, however, means that prospective parents with kidney problems have good chances of conceiving and achieving a healthy pregnancy and birth. Even women with kidney transplants have had babies successfully and go on to have more than one child. These mothers will probably need more prenatal and renal visits to maximize their chances of successful pregnancy.

Diabetes

Non-insulin dependent diabetics can be successfully treated during pregnancy with diet and oral medication. Some patients may require the temporary use of insulin, since pregnancy can disturb insulin levels. Diabetic patients who are stable and following their recommended treatments are as fertile as the rest of the population, but they are more at risk at all stages of pregnancy. A successful pregnancy relies on careful control of diet and adequate levels of nutrition. Morning sickness may complicate insulin control, and you should seek your doctor's advice if you suffer from this. There are also several complementary therapies, such as acupuncture, and remedies such as ginger that can help without unwanted side-effects.

HIV/AIDS and pregnancy

Unprotected sex can expose either partner to a number of diseases, some of which cause infertility, while others are potentially fatal. HIV/AIDS is of particular concern because treatments have not yet been developed that completely halt the progress of this life-threatening virus. Meanwhile, transmission rates among all sections of society—men, women, and children—continue to grow.

The good news is that HIV survivors have shown that in many ways the disease can be treated like other chronic, life-threatening illnesses. Many couples, with one or both partners HIV positive, are choosing to conceive. With the support of health care professionals and self-help groups, they are achieving healthy pregnancies and births.

However, people living with HIV have a higher level of health risk. If you are in this situation and thinking about conception, you may want to consider a number of questions. They include the practical and emotional impacts on your lives, how best to achieve a healthy conception, what forms of medical and complementary treatments to consider, and which birth method is safest.

Should we have an HIV/AIDS test? If you have any reason to believe that either you or your partner may have become infected with the AIDS virus, seek professional medical advice and have an HIV test now, before you conceive. Prompt action can improve your chances of a healthy conception. It will also provide you with access to the best advice.

The test itself is fairly simple—a straightforward blood test looking for the presence of HIV antibodies—but your response to it may be very complex, impacting on your sense of self, your relationships, work, and social life. The test itself is always preceded by counseling, but

a positive result is likely to be a severe shock, and it may be some time before you consider whether or not to go ahead and conceive.

How can we maintain a loving relationship? In the event of a positive result, you will be given advice on how to avoid spreading the virus, including using barrier contraceptive methods during sex. The virus resides in blood and cannot survive for long outside these warm, damp conditions. For this reason, it is not usually transmitted by touch, and holding hands, embraces, and massage are all quite safe.

It is important for you both to maintain an optimum level of wellbeing to keep the virus from developing into full AIDS. Walking, swimming, and other everyday leisure activities are all good for you. High nutritional levels are a must, and the ideas contained in Chapter 2 (Boosting your fertility) will also help improve your immune system. The complementary techniques described in Chapter 4 may help you to relax and deal with the additional pressures that living with HIV can bring.

Should we try to conceive? Couples may find that only one of them has the virus, and the most important practical issue is how to conceive without spreading the infection. Unprotected sex runs the double risk of transmitting the disease to your partner and to your unborn child, but there are ways of reducing this risk.

Although normal touch will not transmit the virus, women who are planning to get pregnant should be careful about caring for a partner with HIV/AIDS. Sperm does carry the virus, but your doctor may be able to arrange for the sperm to be "washed," although this technique is not yet widely available. An alternative may be to consider donor insemination (see pages 126–129).

For women with the virus, the safest option is to self-inseminate with your partner's sperm to avoid the risk of his catching the virus. This is a procedure which can be easily carried out at home, using simple equipment. Timing is critical for women with the HIV virus—the risk of transmission to your future child can be reduced if you conceive when you are free from symptoms or from other infections.

Will pregnancy bring on full AIDS?

Becoming pregnant when HIV-positive does not increase the chance of the mother-to-be developing full AIDS. One of the key factors is your health at the time of conception. Depending on the particular circumstances, the anti-HIV/AIDS drug, AZT (zidovudine),

can help some mothers-to-be control the virus during pregnancy, while improving their health and that of their child.

Will our child inherit the virus?

While HIV infection may pass between mother and child during pregnancy, this doesn't mean that the child will go on to develop AIDS. Most babies born to mothers with HIV are not infected, but the risk is particularly high at birth, and you will need to discuss the birth options available to reduce it. You may be advised not to breastfeed, since the infection can pass through mother's milk, but the benefits of breast milk may outweigh the risks.

This white blood cell is infected with the HIV virus, visible as pink dots budding from the cell. In some countries, HIV testing is now recommended for all pregnant women to reduce the risk of infecting unborn children.

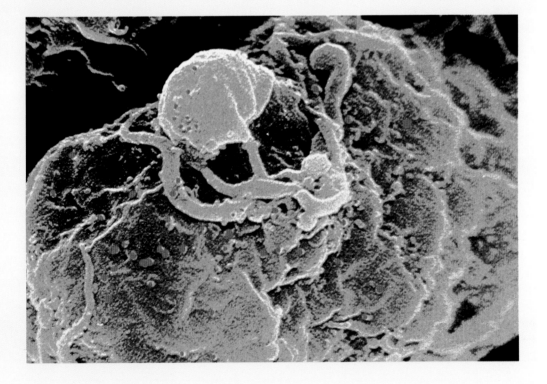

Chapter two

Boost your fertility

Nature supplies our needs in abundance: for every young tree a hundred seeds lie dormant on the forest floor. Likewise, men generate millions more than the single sperm needed to fertilize an egg, and women are born with a ready storehouse of eggs.

In recent years there have been more and more stories about declining sperm counts and fertility problems. Typically, these focus on the number of sperm or eggs instead of their quality; on mechanical interventions instead of natural solutions. In reality, these problems affect very few of us, but they can alarm otherwise healthy couples.

The fertility process has phases of growth and maturity followed by rest, which take place continuously on a microscopic level. Whatever your concerns, working with your natural cycles to boost your fertility will improve your health and increase your chances of a healthy conception. You will feel relaxed and prepared for pregnancy, fit for the physical and emotional demands of parenthood.

The approach to preconceptional care outlined in this book has been developed by clinicians working closely with couples over many years. It is reassuring to know that this method has a high success rate, even with couples in so-called "problem" groups. Preconceptional care helps people who have experienced difficulty conceiving, as well as those who simply want to give their future family the best possible start in life. It offers safe, effective advice, caring for parents and delivering healthy babies without complications.

The moment of fertilization, when a sperm fuses with an egg, marks the beginning of a human life. Once one sperm has managed to penetrate the egg, the surface changes to prevent other sperm from entering.

Boost your fertility in five easy steps

This chapter looks at the five steps to a healthy conception and shows how a natural, holistic approach can help to improve your fertility and build up your natural vitality. Rebalancing takes time as you change old habits, improve your diet, and develop new routines. Personal benefits will be evident in reduced premenstrual syndrome and regular ovulatory cycles. Your fertility levels will be rising at the same time, improving your chances of a healthy conception.

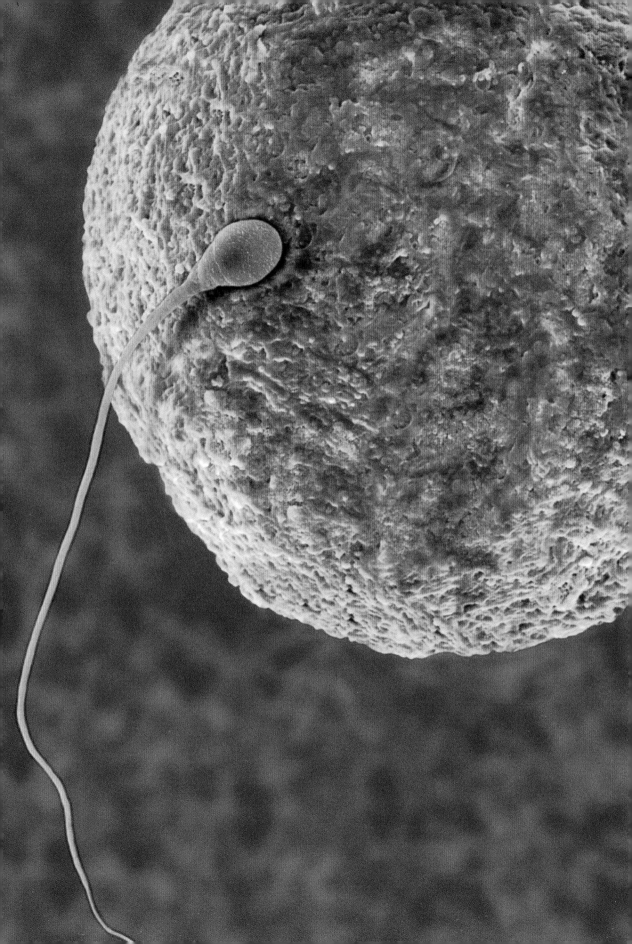

Five steps to a healthy conception

Boosting your fertility consists of five practical steps to detoxify and strengthen your physical system and balance your mind, body, and spirit. These steps are designed to make sure you work alongside your body's own fertility cycles. For men, sperm develops and matures over three months, so boosting your fertility in that time will mean that your sperm gets the best possible nutrients. For women, it is just as important to regularize and smooth the passage of eggs into the womb and to create a nourishing environment for the fertilized egg, when you achieve your goal of conception.

Step one: Adapt your lifestyle

- Write your lifestyle diary (see page 40) and your family medical history questionnaire.
- Be realistic about your tobacco, alcohol, or drug consumption.
- Prepare to make personal lifestyle changes in key areas.
- Improve your nutrition.

Step two: Improve your wellbeing

- Have a general health check, plus any specific diagnostic tests.
- Find ways to reduce medication for long-standing conditions.
- Have a dental checkup and all the treatment you need.
- Treat infections and problems identified in tests.

Step three: Detoxify your system

- Filter your water and aim to drink four full glasses during the day.
- Cut down on caffeine-based drinks and the snacks you eat with them.
- Add more fresh food, containing as few additives as possible, to your diet.
- Take recommended vitamin and mineral supplements.

Step four: Improve your environment

- Avoid contact with toxic chemicals in your home and work place.
- Discuss your concerns with your clinician and employers.
- Complete any renovations and redecoration, and ventilate your home thoroughly.
- Use plants to neutralize a static environment.

Step five: Relax and stay positive

- Learn to share your concerns and banish stress.
- Find ways of relaxing together.
- Start a gentle exercise routine.
- Maintain a balance between your goal of conception and a contented life.

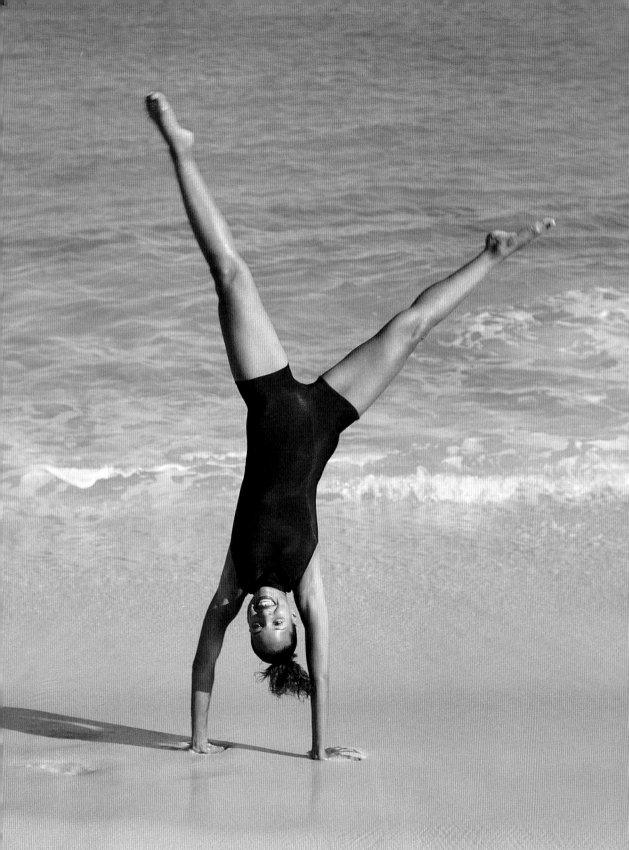

Step one: Adapt your lifestyle

Making changes to your lifestyle can be a series of small steps rather than a great leap. Don't try to do everything at once. Break down your targets into manageable actions and chart your progress, giving yourselves treats to keep your motivation going.

Begin a diary of your daily activities, including eating habits and sleeping patterns (see the example on page 132). Assess how healthy you really are and identify where your priorities lie.

Note down your concerns about possible hazards at work or at home. Look at the way you travel to work and the amount of driving you do. Build up a realistic picture of your lifestyle and note points such as how much exercise you take, how often you eat fresh fruit, how much alcohol you drink. Moderate alcohol intake has some beneficial health effects, but our perceptions of "moderate" are highly subjective. Occasional drinking "binges" are the worst of all for your health.

The lifestyle diary, combined with your personal and family medical history, will help you spot hidden health links and patterns. For example, you might notice that a facial rash has been caused by a combination of stress and milk allergy. Once you have identified links and recognized the need for change, you can break free of old habits.

Set yourselves simple targets, such as buying a water filter or introducing organic milk. Focus on particular areas—get used to taking your vitamin supplements regularly, for example—and adapt your lifestyle at a gentle pace.

By supporting each other, you can adapt your current lifestyle and introduce new routines. Holistic approaches take time, so you won't notice the benefits immediately. These changes, which represent a commitment to your future family, will also benefit you. They not be easy at first, but you do have choices over these areas of your life. If you have had fertility problems in the past, these steps will make a difference. As you recover your natural fertility levels, your appearance and energy will improve, too.

Remember to review all areas of your life. You may find that an activity you take for granted, such as eating late at night, sleeping on an old bed or regularly working through your lunchbreak, could be having a negative effect on your energy levels. Try breaking these bad habits and experience the benefits.

Lifestyle changes
Tell your friends and relatives that you are making changes. Friendships and family are important, but the health of your future child is vital. Explain what it means to you and ask them to respect your desire for a smoke-free home or to drink less alcohol when you go out for the evening.

Key lifestyle changes

One: Eliminate tobacco

- Active and passive smoking harms your health and that of your future children. Pregnant women are particularly vulnerable and can pass on breathing problems to their children.
- Smoking slows down your ability to conceive and may reduce sperm quality. It is linked to fallopian tube blockages and can increase complications in pregnancy, including miscarriage.
- Smoking is linked to many life-threatening diseases. If you cut down now, avoid other smokers, and stop altogether as soon as you can, your chances of a healthy conception could be the same as those of current non-smokers.

Two: Cut down alcohol

- More than two drinks a day will affect your fertility and can ruin your enjoyment of a close physical relationship. Even "social drinking" can cause immediate and irreversible nutrient deficiencies in the fetus.
- Alcohol is one of the most common causes of male impotence and sterility. It causes sperm abnormalities and reduces testosterone levels. In women, it is linked to miscarriage, stillbirth, and physical abnormalities.
- Alcohol will reduce your ability to conceive; it depletes parental nutrient levels, which are linked to growth, system development, and consequent behavioral difficulties in children.
- Reduce your alcohol intake to a sensible level now. If either of you suffers from yeast-linked conditions, such as candida, your clinician may advise you to cut out alcohol completely for a time.

Three: Reduce medication and recreational drugs

- If you use medication that affects fertility, ask your clinician to check each item and take advice on their reduction.
- With medical supervision, seek alternative methods of treatment, where possible, to help you reduce medication and wean yourself off addictive substances.
- Complementary health care, an improved diet, and nutritional supplements can help you avoid recurrence of migraines and epilepsy and improve diabetes.
- The temporary "highs" from recreational drugs are just not worth the negative effects on your libido and fertility.

Four: Avoid environmental toxins

- Work within health and safety guidelines at all times: avoid harmful situations as far as possible and reduce potential hazards at home and in the work place.
- Remember that even supposedly "safe" substances may have harmful effects on your fertility and pregnancy.

Step two: Improve your wellbeing

To conceive a healthy baby you need to be physically healthy. Even before conception occurs, your bodies demand nutrients from you in order to energize and nourish the egg and sperm on their journey into the womb.

Any infections or nutritional deficiencies you have when you conceive will affect the DNA of your future child. They will also reduce your own energy levels just when you need them to cope with pregnancy and childbirth. This doesn't apply just to women—men are also affected by the demands made on them and their partners during pregnancy and when a new child arrives. Bringing a baby into the world probably demands more preparation than running a marathon!

A good partner in this phase of preparation is your ob-gyn. Explain your plans to prepare for conception and your desire to use an holistic approach, and ask for advice on the tests available to check your fertility, infection, and nutrition levels. If necessary, your doctor can prescribe medication to clear up infections and help you reduce long-standing prescription drugs. For some conditions, such as migraine, diabetes, or epilepsy, an improved nutritional balance can help reduce the amount of medication you need. You may be recommended to a fertility or nutritional expert who has particular experience in holistic approaches to fertility. If you go direct to a specialist, make sure you keep your family physician informed. Your medical records will contain valuable clinical information that can assist your planned conception.

Discuss any worries you have about your situation at work with your clinician and gain his support in communicating with your employers. By working together this way, you will safeguard your health and fertility.

What do doctors mean by "infertility"?

Infertility is defined as the inability to achieve pregnancy within a year (see page 82). This is why clinicians often advise couples to "go away and keep on trying" for a year or longer before they counsel medical infertility treatments.

It is estimated that up to one in ten couples are "subfertile," which means that we are all likely to know at least one couple in this situation. Subfertile couples are those who have a reduced level of fertility, due to factors in either partner. Of these, many can be helped to conceive and deliver a healthy baby without the need for artificial hormone or other medical treatments. You can

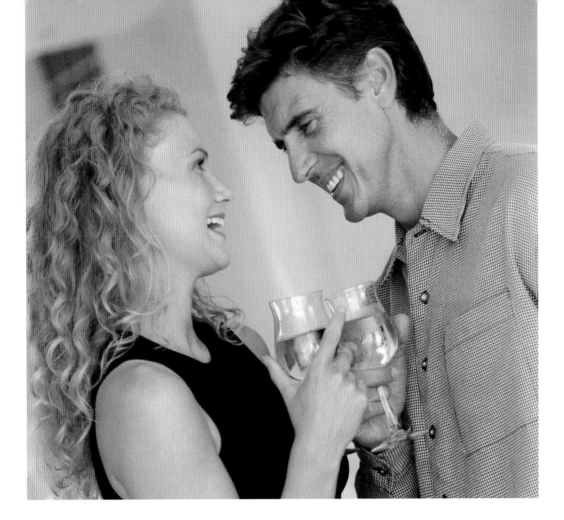

often avoid unwanted side-effects and possible health risks by using a natural approach.

Causes of subfertility vary, but poor diet, chemically-contaminated water and food, and harmful substances in everyday products are typical. Whatever the cause, detoxifying and rebalancing the body will help. Use your time wisely by taking steps to cleanse your system and boost your wellbeing. Detoxing your system can reduce your waiting time while improving your overall health.

Temporary infertility is not necessarily a sign of total sterility. Many couples previously described as "infertile" have gone on to have healthy children using the approach in this book. Take positive action to boost your fertility—now!

Contraception

The use of some forms of contraception, such as the pill or an intrauterine device (IUD), can cause a fertility delay of up to two years. The pill raises the background level of hormones in the body. These need to drop and a normal menstrual cycle reestablished, before conception can take place.

A few glasses of wine at a social occasion may seem harmless, but alcohol can reduce your fertility and cause damage to the fetus. For the sake of your future children's health, reduce your alcohol intake now.

In the case of IUDs, particularly those made of copper, there is a possible double effect of high levels of copper (which kills sperm) and localized infection in the uterus to overcome before conception can take place.

You may to choose to use barrier contraceptive methods during your countdown to conception. This will typically be a combination of the condom and the cap. Avoid lubricating gels or spermicidal creams containing nonoxonyl 9, since this ingredient kills sperm and is associated with cystitis and other infections that directly or indirectly affect fertility. Some couples may prefer to use natural family planning (NFP) instead of barrier methods, but this approach should be properly taught if it is to be effective. As your fertility awareness increases (see Chapter 3), you will get to know which barrier method suits different stages of your cycle best.

Typical diagnostic tests

Before your clinicians recommend any course of medical treatment or nutritional supplements, they will want to give you a thorough health check. In addition to asking you for your family medical history—going back to both sets of grandparents if possible—they may ask detailed supplementary questions.

They will also propose an astonishing array of tests—some of which might not be familiar to you. Blood and urine samples give an indication of your general state of health; fertility tests will check sperm levels and condition (explained more fully in Chapter 3). Women will be advised to have a smear test, and men will generally be given a prostate test.

You could also be asked for sweat and hair samples. Analyzed in a laboratory, these samples help your clinician to check on the presence of heavy metals in your system over a period of time, as well as to determine your current nutrient levels. It is critical that tests identify all your vitamin and mineral deficiencies, as well as the presence of any toxic metals.

Based on your test results, you will be advised on the most appropriate treatment and diet, plus the combination of vitamin and mineral supplements to suit your special health needs. Whatever course of treatment you are prescribed, the principle will be to diagnose, treat, and then re-test to check the effectiveness of the treatment.

Boosting your fertility—men

Male infertility typically occurs for one of three reasons, which can be confirmed or ruled out by sperm tests:

- Poor sperm quality—sperm that lack vigor, clump together, or are misshapen.
- Low numbers of sperm—sperm are not being produced regularly in the body.
- Poor environment—maturing sperm lack nourishment and energy.

Remember, even if you are one of the one in twenty men with a reduced sperm count, there is a lot you can do to put the situation right. Get rid of any infections or lingering ailments

Boosting male fertility

Cut out hazards

Cigarette smoking
- Depletes vitamin C absorption.
- Produces estrogenlike female hormones.

Alcohol
- Causes zinc depletion that interferes with normal sexual development and reduces sperm count and testosterone levels.

Chemicals in food, water, and environment
- Diminish ability to absorb trace minerals, notably zinc, manganese, and iron.
- May cause birth defects.
- May cause cancer.

Food additives
- Injure chromosomes and genes.
- May cause birth defects.
- May cause allergies.

Reap the benefits

Vitamin C
- Aids in the absorption of iron.
- Provides oxidants to semen.
- Prevents sperm "clumping."
- Improves vitality.

Zinc
- Is important for cell division.
- Is vital for the development of primary and secondary sexual characteristics.
- Is necessary for sperm creation.

Trace minerals critical to health and fertility:
- Zinc (see above).
- Manganese for muscle tone.
- Magnesium and potassium for sperm motility.

Unprocessed natural foods
- Improve absorption of nutritional elements.
- Improve sperm quality and genetic inheritance.
- Reduce likelihood of allergies.

and give yourself at least three months to boost your fertility—that's how long it takes to develop mature, vigorous sperm.

For men, zinc, magnesium, and B-complex vitamins help sperm development. Where tests show sperm "clumping" (agglutination), vitamin C is a simple and inexpensive solution to the problem. Supplements of vitamin E and selenium help sperm quality, levels, and motility (strength and movement).

Take positive steps to increase your fertility and improve your general vitality by identifying and then cutting out the major

Boosting female fertility

Cut out the hazards

Cigarette smoking
- Depletes vitamin C.
- Causes cancer.
- Slows down your ability to conceive.
- Is linked to fallopian tube blockages.
- Increases complications in pregnancy.
- May lead to a child with a low birth weight.
- Passes on health problems to your child.

Alcohol
- Flushes vital nutrients such as trace minerals, which are required from the very moment of conception, out of the system.

Chemicals in food, water, and environment
- Diminish ability to absorb trace minerals such as zinc and iron.
- May cause birth defects.
- May cause cancer.

Food additives
- May injure chromosomes and genes.
- May cause birth defects.
- May cause allergies.

Reap the benefits

Vitamin C
- Aids in the absorption of iron.
- Improves vitality.
- Speeds up your countdown to conception.
- Helps you have an easier pregnancy.
- Improves the health of your future child.

Trace minerals
- Improve fertility levels.
- Reduce birth defects.
- Improve the health of your future child.

Zinc and iron
- High zinc levels help avoid miscarriage.
- Good iron levels reduce anemia, depression, and headaches.

Unprocessed natural foods
- Improve nutritional absorption.
- Improve genetic inheritance.
- Reduce likelihood of allergies.

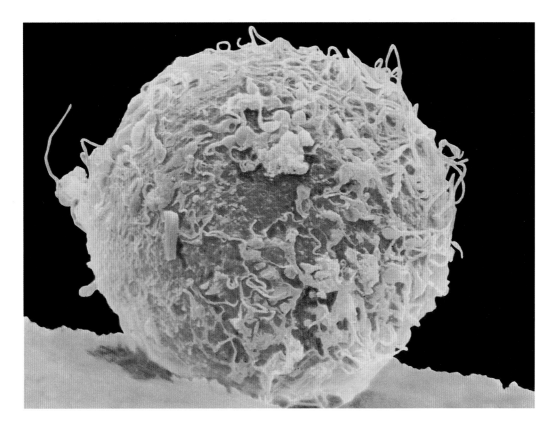

hazards noted in the chart on page 45. You will reap the benefits personally, and pass on the best possible DNA to your offspring.

Boosting your fertility—women

Female fertility problems are typically linked to ovulation, menstruation, or blockages in the fallopian tubes. Women are born with a set number of immature eggs stored in the ovaries. These eggs cannot be replaced in the way sperm is. Damage to your eggs or ovaries will reduce their number and, therefore, your chances of conception, but may not render you infertile.

Deficiencies in zinc, magnesium, the B-complex vitamins, and essential fatty acids (EFAs) have all been linked to fertility problems, difficulties in pregnancy, and postnatal depression as well as to restlessness and failure to thrive in babies. By taking positive steps now, you can avoid these problems from the start of your pregnancy.

There's plenty you can do to help yourself, such as cutting out smoking and increasing your vitamin-C intake. Boosting your fertility will reduce problems associated with menstruation, such as premenstrual tension, as well as tiredness and water retention.

The survival of the fittest—only one of the many millions of sperm released in an ejaculation may penetrate an egg. This colored scanning electron micrograph shows a number of sperm, visible as slender yellow structures, clustered around an egg.

Step three: Detoxify your system

Cleansing your system will improve your intake and absorption of vital nutrients. The loss of just one—even for a short time during early pregnancy—can be crucial. Common problems such as miscarriage, premature birth, and low birth weight can all be avoided by paying careful attention to diet both before conception takes place and during pregnancy.

Purify your water

Some drinking water is contaminated with chemicals and metals that may affect your fertility. There are distinct regional differences, depending on local water supplies and the use of particular chemicals. Tap water can contain lead or cadmium contamination from plumbing connections or pipes, or aluminum from the treatment process.

Chlorine, pesticide, and fertilizer residues may also be present. This can be because not all the pesticide or fertilizer sprayed on crops is taken up. The chemicals then combine with organic matter in the soil or leach into surface or ground water. Many farmers are now looking at ways of reducing their use of chemicals or are converting to organic methods. You may be able to have your water tested by the water company, who should list the contaminants and tell you whether it meets standards.

Water filters are a simple and inexpensive way to improve your water supply and remove contaminants. Both filter jugs and faucet connections have been shown to lower levels of metals and chemicals substantially, while improving the taste. If further tests show that your water is still contaminated after filtering, use bottled spring water. Aim to drink 2 pints of pure water every day as part of your countdown to conception. The benefits are two-fold: you will reduce your intake of toxins and help to flush out those already in your system.

Improve your diet

Our ability to reproduce is extremely sensitive to the availability and quality of food. This is equally true of our desire and potency for lovemaking. The effects of excessive weight gain or loss on fertility are known; less well understood are the minute-to-minute metabolic changes that take place in the body and can also affect fertility.

You might assume that you eat a "good diet," simply by following the habits in which you were brought up. Sadly, with the quality of many foods declining, what was good

To detoxify your system
- Reduce intake of unwanted additives and contaminants.
- Remove toxins that are currently in your system
- Improve and sustain your intake of nutrients.

for our parents may not be as nutritious now. Some vitamin deficiencies are linked to poor dietary habits, such as high alcohol consumption, regular use of white sugar or flour products, or poor protein intake. In addition, you may lead a busy life, snatching prepared meals or snacking on junk food with little or no nutritional value.

Food additives—often unnecessary coloring, preservatives, and sweeteners—add to the cocktail of ingredients not required by the body. Aluminum, for example, is often contained in milk substitutes just to help pouring qualities. It is feared that many of these additives could injure our genetic code during sperm and egg maturation. They could affect the health of unborn children at their most vulnerable point of development.

Regular meals, including a healthy breakfast, will make a positive difference. Avoid refined products made with white flour and sugar or saturated fats. Cut down on your consumption of tea and coffee. Be careful about the way you store and cook food. Leafy vegetables, rhubarb, and apples, for example, are particularly prone to "leaching" metal from aluminum pans so avoid using them with these foods.

Give added zest to your life by switching to fresh foods with as few additives as possible. Make a priority of building up to five portions of fruit and vegetables a day. Replace essential nutrients through a varied diet that stimulates your appetite. Breaking old eating habits and improving your diet may be a challenge, but the physical benefits will soon be apparent.

Food intolerances

Many people now suffer from food intolerances or allergies. Common symptoms include migraines, headaches, sneezing fits, asthma, and rashes, even irritable bowel syndrome. So-called "psychological" or behavioral symptoms, such as tiredness and depression, may also be linked to allergies. The good news is that these problems typically improve once the allergic trigger has been found and eliminated. Typical causes include artificial food coloring, cow's milk, chocolate, caffeine, wheat, oranges, eggs, peanuts, and sugar.

There are also increasing problems with "subclinical" nutritional problems. This is where poor food quality may not be enough to make you ill but could affect your fertility. Keep a food diary, check the quality of your diet with your clinician, and take steps to improve deficiencies.

There is also a possibility of a combination factor, where one allergy trigger may interact with another—you are particularly likely to be susceptible when you are under stress. It is important to consider food sensitivities in combination with other factors. Do this under the guidance of a professional nutritionist: don't simply remove foods from your diet.

The benefits of organic produce

Allergic reactions can be caused by additives or pesticides on food, rather than by the food itself. With some fruit and cereal crops treated up to 15 times, residues may be above safe levels. Avoid these toxins by switching to organic fruit and vegetables, and free-range eggs and meat. Drink organic milk to avoid the high estrogen levels found in intensively farmed herds. Even homegrown fruit and vegetables may be contaminated by industrial dust. If you do live near a factory site or road, always wash your own produce thoroughly. Homegrown fresh fruit, for example, provides an excellent regular source of vitamin C, but always wash the skin well before eating.

Organically grown foods store a far greater concentration of nutrients than ordinary crops, and the concentration of toxic metals is lower. This provides the double benefit of improving nutrition and reducing toxins. Try to make sure that the food you buy is as fresh as possible. The vitamin content of vegetables and fruit, even if organic, deteriorates with age.

Organic foods and milk are now widely available. For some couples, price is an important deciding factor when shopping; fortunately some supermarkets and local delivery services are now selling organic foods at prices comparable to standard lines, making them increasingly affordable.

Vegetarian, vegan, or dairy-free diets

Meat is not essential for a healthy conception or pregnancy since all of the nutritional benefits of meat can also be found in other foods. A typical western diet contains fairly high levels of meat, which can cause multiple health problems. Meat not from organic sources can contain antibiotics and, in some cases, growth hormones.

If you have a milk sensitivity, you might be advised to avoid dairy products or to switch to organic sources. Organic milk products are, however, a source of vitamins and minerals, including folic acid.

You may, by personal preference, avoid meat and dairy products altogether in your diet. All the nutritional benefits

Vegetables provide pro-vitamin A, inositol, folic acid, and vitamin C. Because vitamin C is destroyed by cooking, eat vegetables raw where possible. Sprouted seeds and green leafy vegetables provide pro-vitamin A, vitamins B2, B5, B12, C, E, and K, essential fatty acids (EFAs), PABA, choline, and folic acid. Sprouted seeds are also a good source of calcium, necessary for the essential moment of fertilization .

Fruit provides pro-vitamin A as well as vitamins E, C, and inositol. Most fruits are best eaten raw.

Wholegrains, wheatgerm, beans, and legumes provide vitamins E, B1, B2, B3, B5, B6, and B12, PABA, biotin, inositol, choline, and folic acid. Oils, seeds, and nuts provide vitamins B1, B2, B3, B6, and E, essential fatty acids (EFAs), and folic acid. Unrefined, cold-pressed oils are the best types. Peanuts may cause allergic reactions in some people.

Fish and fish oils, particularly cod liver oil, provide vitamins A and D, essential fatty acids (EFAs), B2 (riboflavin), B3 (niacin), biotin, choline, and B12.

Organic free-range eggs provide pro-vitamin A and vitamins B2, B5, B12, and D, as well as choline and biotin. Raw egg white destroys biotin, and pregnant women should avoid undercooked eggs completely because of the risk of salmonella.

can be found by switching to other foods as long as you maintain a healthy nutritional balance. Green leaves, grains, and seeds can, for example, be even better sources of calcium than milk. The important point to remember is that reducing junk food, eating a wholesome diet, and using fewer refined products such as white sugar and bleached flour are probably the most important steps you can take toward a healthy conception.

Vitamins and minerals

Vitamins and minerals are present in our food in minute quantities and are essential for our metabolism. Deficiencies are known to cause disease, affect fertility levels, and have links to birth defects.

However, vitamins and minerals do need to be regularly replaced—either through improving your diet or by taking supplements. Storing and cooking food carefully avoids destroying vitamins: for example, milk left in sunlight will lose its vitamin B2 and overcooking food destroys vitamins B and C. So unless your diet is composed of fresh, organic foods— preferably served raw—it is likely that it will have reduced vitamin levels. You may also find that an apparently good food source is contaminated with pesticide or other residues.

Identify nutritional sources of vitamins and minerals, and use them to restore natural levels in your body. Look out for sources of organic foods such as wheat bran, leafy vegetables, eggs, dairy, and meat products—particularly liver. (Variety meat contains large amounts of toxins if it is not organic.)

Certain vitamins and minerals may be recommended by your clinician to cleanse your system of heavy metals. Particular foods may be indicated, such as legumes that "bind" with heavy metals and carry them out of the body. Food supplements, such as blue-green algae, are also used to neutralize and remove toxins, or to improve your immune system.

You could also be deficient in important nutrients, vital for optimum fertility. Smoking will deplete your natural reserves of vitamin C, lowering your energy and immunity to illness. Caffeine, alcohol, and even stress are known to deplete magnesium and vitamin B levels. Mercury used in fillings for teeth (amalgam) is connected with fertility problems.

Vitamin and mineral supplements are now recognized as important for improving your fertility and helping you prepare for a healthy conception. Medical evidence shows that supplements—including those taken before conception— improve the health of both you and your baby. You can detoxify

Folic acid

Folic acid is critical for good functioning of the nervous system. It supports red blood cell formation and helps produce DNA and RNA. It also metabolizes sugar and amino acids, and helps manufacture antibodies. Essential for the metabolism of zinc and supplements, folic acid helps avoid depression, dizziness, and anemia.

High levels of folic acid must be present from the moment of conception. It supports the tremendous cell growth in the early stages of pregnancy and is important for the development of organs and tissues in the fetus from the very start, before some women know they are pregnant. The recommended daily allowance of folic acid is 200 micrograms.

your body and replace lost nutrients through vitamin and mineral supplements.

Fat-soluble and water-soluble vitamins

Vitamins are complicated substances themselves, often made up of a number of components. They divide into two main groups:

- Fat-soluble vitamins (A, D, E, and K) and the essential fatty acids (EFAs are not strictly vitamins, but an important nutritional component).
- Water-soluble vitamins (B-complex and C).

The fat-soluble vitamins are stored in the body—beneficial when you are planning to conceive. In early pregnancy, the fetus will draw on the accumulated stores, even when you cannot be sure you have conceived.

Water-soluble vitamins are not stored in the body and are easily lost through cooking—hence the need to increase your consumption of fresh, raw foods. These vitamins must be replaced regularly through diet or supplementation.

B-complex vitamins are lost at times of stress and infection, and are in greater demand during pregnancy and lactation. For this reason, it is important to recognize stressful situations as times when you will need extra supplements.

Vitamin and mineral combinations target your areas of deficiency and speed up the fertility boosting process, interacting in complex biochemical processes. The B-complex vitamins work together and should not be taken in isolation. You may be advised to take a combination of vitamins and minerals, depending on your particular needs. Your recommended daily intake will also change during your countdown to conception and into pregnancy.

Taking food supplements that promote fertility requires careful analysis and individual guidance, since vitamins or minerals in isolation can cause problems—you need the correct combination. Your clinician will assess your needs carefully to make sure the quantities you take are no higher than necessary.

It will be some time before you get into the habit of taking nutritional supplements, but it is important to establish a routine. Many are not stored in your body, but are needed on a regular basis. Take them as recommended and at the times of day specified. Your aim is to achieve a balance: never exceed the recommended dose—you may do more harm than good—or try to rush your program of supplements.

PABA (Para-amino Benzoic Acid)
PABA is part of all folic acids and is required for their formation. A factor in the vitamin B complex—known as a "vitamin within a vitamin"—it is involved in the breaking down of protein and the formation of red blood cells. PABA also stimulates intestinal bacteria to help them make folic acid, which in turn makes pantothenic acid. A common ingredient in ultraviolet screens, PABA helps to protect the skin. There is no recommended daily allowance, but the suggested daily supplement level (see page 55) is 30–100 milligrams.

The benefits of vitamin supplements

Vitamin	Good for you
Vitamin A	For healthy eyes, skin, and gums. Builds resistance, promotes growth, and aids tissue repair. Linked to improving reproductive problems.
Vitamin B1 (Thiamin)	For growth. B1 metabolizes carbohydrates to glucose for energy, or to fat for storage. Water soluble and heat sensitive, so it is easily lost in cooking. Especially important for nerves.
Vitamin B2 (Riboflavin)	Linked with formation of liver enzymes and the use of oxygen in the metabolism of carbohydrates, fats, and proteins stored in the liver. Important for protection against toxins, as an antioxidant, and for detoxing
Vitamin B3 (Niacin)	Assists in the utilization of energy and the creation of sex hormones. Helps develop proper nerve function. Deficiency associated with pellagra, a disease causing diarrhea, skin problems, and dementia.
Vitamin B5 (Pantothenic acid)	Helps the immune system. Required by every cell in the body to metabolize sugar and fat. Helps the body withstand stress.
Vitamin B6 (Pyridoxine)	Helps metabolize proteins, amino acids, sugars, fatty acids, and some minerals. Involved in the manufacture of red blood cells, antibodies, hormones, and enzymes. Essential for growth and the synthesis of RNA and DNA. Helps utilize minerals such as zinc, magnesium, and manganese.
Vitamin B12 (Cobalamin)	Essential for the function of all cells, particularly hormones and red blood cells. Is used with folic acid in the making of choline, RNA, and DNA.
Vitamin C	The "healing vitamin," vital for healthy skin, bones, and muscles. Protects from viruses and allergies. Improves resistance to toxins such as lead or dangerous drugs and promotes healing after infection, surgery, or injury.
Vitamin D	Needed for healthy growth of bones and teeth. Aids absorption of calcium and magnesium. Can be made from sunlight on skin.
Vitamin E	Has a wide protective effect: preventing scarring or healing abrasions after childbirth; improves muscle function.
Essential fatty acids (EFAs) - including linoleic, linoleni, & arachidonic acids.	Vital to the normal development of nervous and immune systems. Necessary for the absorption of vitamins A, E, D, and K, as well as trace elements. Affect all cells and systems in the body and are used to make sex and adrenal hormones.
Vitamin K	Normally made in the healthy intestine and essential for blood clotting.

Good for healthy conception	RDA[†]
May help to prevent birth defects, avoid infections, and develop a good appetite. Creates the male hormones needed for reproduction.	800 micrograms
Helps to avoid mental health problems, poor concentration and memory, fatigue and irritability. Helps correct sterility and infertility, reduces vomiting, improves appetite, and thus birth weight. Helps avoid stillbirth.	1.1 milligrams
Deficiency must be avoided at all costs, since it has serious effects in pregnancy. Supplementation will produce healthy eyes, skin, lips, nails, and hair.	1.3 milligrams
Prevents headaches, tension, nervousness, and more serious mental health problems. Helps prevent birth defects such as cleft palate.	15 milligrams
Supplements will assist in insomnia, depression, and digestive problems, particularly nausea during pregnancy. Deficiencies may contribute to a variety of reproductive problems.	6 milligrams
Linked to sleeplessness and night cramps. Premenstrual syndrome improves with B6 supplements, as do sickness and other pregnancy problems.	1.6 milligrams
Needed for healthy sperm. Improves menstrual difficulties. Helps balance the nervous system, reduce tiredness, and improve skin disorders.	2 micrograms
Deficiency is linked to miscarriage and poor resistance to infections in children. Helps the absorption of iron and is important for overall wellbeing and good mental health.	60 milligrams
Helps prevent birth defects connected with skull, jaw, and face. Supplements will help avoid joint pains and osteoporosis, as well as night cramps, night sweats, and hot flushes.	5 micrograms
Particularly beneficial for sperm development; helps maturing sperm develop flexibility. Prevents miscarriages and eases labor. Helps to reduce labor time and avoid fetal oxygen deficiency.	8 milligrams
Deficiencies linked to male infertility, also a factor in pre-eclampsia and low birth weight. Help allergies, skin problems, heart and circulatory conditions. Particularly useful for regulating ovulation and menstruation.	700mg[‡] (Linseed) 1000mg[‡] (Fish oil) 500mg[‡] (Evening primrose)
Deficiencies could create birth problems, but are normally avoided through a healthy diet.	65 micrograms[‡]

[†] **Recommended Daily Allowances** obtained from the USDA.
[‡] Where no RDA exists a "Suggested Adult Daily Supplement Level" is proposed.
These are guidelines only. Each individual's needs differ, so check with your clinician.

The benefits of mineral supplements

Mineral	Good for you
Calcium	Well known for its role in developing healthy bones and teeth. Has an important function in protecting against allergies and viruses. Controls blood clotting and assists in muscle growth and function.
Chromium	Vital for fat and carbohydrate metabolism and the production of energy. Important for those suffering from diabetes and high blood pressure.
Copper	Assists in brain development, as well as in the formation of bones, nerves, and connective tissue. Essential in the production of RNA. Excess may cause depression and behavioral problems.
Iodine	An essential element for normal growth. Necessary for the production of substances for physical and mental development, and for overall wellbeing.
Iron	Vital for the manufacture of hemoglobin (the substance in red blood cells that transports oxygen around the body). Helps the digestion of protein, energy production, and in respiration. Anemia is associated with diets lacking in iron and containing excess white flour and sugar.
Magnesium	Needed for producing and transferring energy, for proper nerve and muscle relaxation. Associated with the production of many enzymes and essential for bone metabolism; deficiency can lead to spasms, jumpiness, and irritability.
Manganese	Important for the reproductive system, although its exact function is not fully understood. Also needed for bone growth, nerve function, and enzyme reactions.
Phosphorus	Typically, abundant in the body and works with calcium, particularly in bone development and maintenance. Also plays a part in every chemical reaction in the body.
Potassium	Necessary for growth, good nerve and muscle functioning. Helps maintain fluid levels in the body and with the take-up of enzymes.
Selenium	Closely associated with vitamin E; is a strong antioxidant, prevents chromosomal damage associated with birth defects. Helps fight infections and assists in cell growth. It will combine with heavy metals, helping to detoxify the body.
Zinc	Vital for the maintenance of the immune system, hormone levels, and sperm development. An important component of semen and necessary to stabilize RNA. Required for the utilization of many enzymes. Helps prevent impotence and increases sperm motility. Increases the size of the sex organs in growing boys.

	RDA[†]
Helps avoid premenstrual problems. Vital for the growth of the fetus and the wellbeing of the mother. Levels must be high before conception is achieved. Eases leg cramps and labor pains, and helps achieve a good birth weight.	800 milligrams
Male diabetics who wish to father a child may be recommended to take chromium supplements. Even a small deficiency may be serious, since chromium is not easily absorbed or stored in the body.	25 micrograms[‡]
Deficiencies are rare, but can lead to infertility. Copper in excess can be toxic to sperm. Copper levels must be balanced at the point of conception, since they will rise naturally during pregnancy.	1.2 milligrams[‡]
Deficiencies are linked to fatigue and a loss of interest in sex, as well as the slow development of sex organs. Supplements during pregnancy help promote mental growth and physical development in children.	150 micrograms
Helps anemia, depression, and headaches. Needed in greater quantity during pregnancy, when red blood cells increase by a third. It should always be given in combination with other nutrients. Taken by itself, it can cause depletion of other essential minerals. Vital for a good birth weight.	15 milligrams
Pregnancy makes a magnesium deficiency worse and is linked to painful contractions and possibly miscarriage. Supplements will help avoid miscarriages, low-birth-weight babies, and premature birth.	280 milligrams
Supplements in combination help improve the sex drive and promote the production of sperm and their delivery mechanisms.	15 milligrams[‡]
Phosphorus assists in important hormonal functions. Deficiency is rare, since it is found in many common whole foods, which are the best source of supplementation. Important for a good birth weight.	800 milligrams[‡]
Deficiency may be caused by some medical treatments or eating too little fruit and vegetables. Related to poor sperm motility.	3,500 milligrams[‡]
Good selenium levels are very important throughout the countdown to conception and into pregnancy. Selenium is also linked to successful breastfeeding and prevention of sudden infant death syndrome.	55 micrograms[‡]
Low zinc levels are associated with menstrual problems, male and female infertility, and low birth weight. Zinc supplements will help avoid miscarriage, improve birth weight, provide children with developed immune systems, and assist in their brain development (and future learning ability).	12 milligrams

[†] **Recommended Daily Allowances** obtained from the USDA.
[‡]Where no RDA exists a "Suggested Adult Daily Supplement Level" is proposed.
These are guidelines only. Each individual's needs differ, so check with your clinician.

Step four: Improve your environment

Improving your environment does not mean becoming a hermit or denying yourself the pleasures of life. However, many of the products and substances we encounter every day may affect our health. In towns and cities, for example, pesticides and fertilizers are used regularly in public spaces, such as parks, golf courses, and sports fields. You may be affected when out walking, jogging, or enjoying your favorite sport. Consider joining, or starting, a local self-help group to lobby for their reduction. By pinpointing problem areas and controlling your own use of possibly harmful products, you are giving yourselves the best possible fertility boost.

It is important to find out about chemicals and toxic metals used in your work place, as well as at home. Toxic substances affect reproduction: in men they can reduce hormone levels, sexual function, and fertility. Toxicity can also lead to defective sperm DNA. This will affect pregnancy and birth outcomes, as well as leading to childhood health risks. Low levels, or combinations, of toxic substances should also be identified and avoided. The best first step is to get informed. The excellent *Natural House Book* by David Pearson (see page 134) is a thorough checklist to help you through the maze of potential hazards, which may be present in your home or in the work place. If you have any concerns about any potential hazards, discuss ways of controlling them with your employers.

Even a simple step such as opening a window—allowing the exchange of air in your office or home—will help. Taking a break for some fresh air will also improve your concentration and memory. Check whether the office air-conditioning system has been "scrubbed" recently: this will reduce transmission of airborne bacteria.

Improving your home and work environment will bring long-term benefits—to you and to your friends and colleagues.

Control these hazards in your home or work place:

- Chemical dust, pesticides, and solvents.
- Electromagnetic emissions from computers, microwaves, and mobile phones.
- Static electricity accumulating in plastic, foam, and rubber materials and in poorly ventilated rooms.
- New carpets or curtains treated with mothproofing chemicals or flame retardants containing antimony.
- Food stored in aluminum or cooked in aluminum pans.

Hazards to avoid
Boost your fertility by reducing or avoiding these common hazards in the home, office, and garden:

- Aluminum cookware
- Antacids (typically used for indigestion)
- Artificially scented cosmetics
- Computer screens
- Copper/brass jewelry
- Electric blanket
- Fly spray
- Foil wrap
- Food additives
- Gas-powered stove or boiler
- Herbicides
- Microwave ovens
- Mothballs
- Paint stripper/wallpaper remover
- Pesticides
- Photocopier
- Plastic foodwrap
- Sunbed
- Canned foods/drinks
- Tuna fish

- Pet-delousing or hygiene products.
- Chemicals in household products such as wallpaper paste, paint, and wooden furniture.
- Lead-contaminated primer, undercoat, or gloss in the paintwork of pre-1960s houses.
- Public parks or spaces recently sprayed with fertilizers or pesticides.
- Gases used in the work place, for example by anesthetists and obstetricians.
- Constant contact with petroleum and diesel fumes or spending long periods behind the wheel of a car, truck, or taxi.

Improve your indoor air quality

Volatile Organic Compounds (VOCs) are a large group of chemicals known to be neurotoxic and to cause fertility problems. They reduce indoor air quality and are associated with sick building syndrome. Like other toxins, they are invisible. VOCs are absorbed by inhalation or through the skin. Effects may be short-lived or can last a lifetime, causing fatigue, lack of concentration, and ear, nose, and throat irritations.

While many products and materials containing VOCs appear to be inert, they are in fact "outgassing" into the atmosphere. Reactions can be triggered when you are involved in building or construction, or if you buy new curtains, carpets, or fiberboard furniture. Increasing the ventilation in your home or office will help disperse VOCs, but you need to allow time to clear the air thoroughly.

Natural detoxifiers

A spider plant is a good companion for your computer, since it will absorb ions and balance humidity. The hairy leaves of the African violet will trap dust and remove toxins. The sharp citrus scent of geranium leaves will freshen your air naturally and encourage you to stay alert while you work.

Where possible, replace your cleaning materials with low-toxic substitutes, which use natural materials and aromas. If you use gas to power your stove or heating, install exhaust fans and have regular safety checks. Over time, replace plastic laminates, vinyl flooring, and particle-board fixtures with solid wood and other natural materials. These actions will benefit your health and the environment.

VOCs are divided into three major categories:

- Pesticides: including fruit and vegetable residues, garden insecticides, and those used on industrial sites.
- Solvents and other volatile chemicals: paint, varnish, wax, sealants, glue, latex backing on carpets, paint stripper, wood preservatives, aerosol sprays, cleaning solutions and disinfectants, air fresheners, personal cosmetics, and stored fuel.
- Indoor contaminants: synthetic fabrics, cleaning materials, pesticides, printing and copying equipment, heating appliances—the latter are typically a problem in airtight buildings with poor ventilation. This category also includes art materials, such as art pens, magic markers, glue and so on. Schools, art rooms, and conference centers may all be sources of exposure.
- Formaldehyde: includes construction materials such as flooring, paneling, paint, wax and glue, upholstery fabrics, cabinets, and furniture made from particle board. It may also be found in newsprint, carbonless-copying paper, and fluids used in dry cleaning.

Toxic chemicals
Approximately 70,000 manufactured chemicals are in use worldwide and not all of these have been tested for toxic effects on human reproduction.

Boost your health and brighten your environment!

Putting plants into your work or home environment isn't just about making visual improvements—houseplants have been shown to detoxify the air we breathe. Plants filter and purify the air by absorbing toxic gases, such as formaldehyde, as well as by converting carbon dioxide into oxygen. You will benefit from fresher air, as well as a more balanced level of humidity. Common houseplants also filter and trap dust, leaving you with a cleaner atmosphere.

Plants need water through their leaves and roots to regulate and modify their humidity and balance ions in the air. We need water to clean our environment and to cleanse our physical systems. In busy, stuffy offices or over-sealed homes with little access to fresh air, we quickly become dehydrated and irritable. Our temperatures rise, our skin prickles, and our nerves fray before we are even aware of our need for water. Yet it is one of the most cleansing, refreshing, and available substances on earth. Keep a bottle of water beside you as you work: drink it and your concentration and performance will improve—and your temper!

Another way of cleansing and beautifying your environment is to harness energy in crystals. The idea of using crystals to dissipate disease was first recorded in an ancient Egyptian papyrus and has recently enjoyed a resurgence of popularity. Astronauts are reported to take quartz crystals into outer space to counteract potential physical and mental disorders created by traveling outside the earth's magnetic field. Many computer professionals keep a piece of amethyst on the top of their VDU to combat atmospheric pollution and reduce the effects of electromagnetic fields.

Textbooks on crystals point out that amethyst is a healing crystal, which promotes contentment and absorbs negativity. Interestingly, it is also associated with the "third eye," the point of focus in the middle of the forehead above the eyebrows (roughly the level of the top of the computer screen). Crystals can be used in every room to inspire, balance, and heal. Rose quartz is a symbol of love; agate and sodalite are believed to improve sleep. Any of these could be used in your bedroom, for example, to calm you and promote inner peace.

Keep your crystals "cleansed" by rinsing them regularly under running water and drying them in the sunshine. This will draw off accumulated negativity and recharge your crystals.

Self-help steps for cutting out chemicals

It is not only single chemicals that are of concern. Combined chemicals also pose a risk, even at low levels, and for this reason they should be avoided.

First, identify the chemical source: such as food, home, work, or public places. Begin a diary and note your contact with potentially hazardous substances. Show it to your clinician and work-place manager. If you have any cause for concern, ask about the available tests for toxic substances.

The next step is to reduce your use of chemicals: check the "ingredients" list on do-it-yourself products or art materials and avoid their use wherever possible.

Finally, detoxify your system: filter your water, improve your diet, and take recommended food supplements when necessary. Low levels of chemicals means a better, healthier, environment for you and your family.

Step five: relax and stay positive

Understand stress factors and fertility

Stress can affect your ability to conceive. Tolerance levels and stress thresholds vary greatly from person to person, which is why we talk about "negative" stress to indicate levels of stimulation that are affecting you. For example, a work-place challenge that stimulates you may be a problem to a colleague. Conversely, what relaxes you might be a bore to someone else.

Vacations can both help and create stress. It is important to take your full entitlement and make sure that at least one break each year is for a whole week. You need time to unwind fully and to enjoy your surroundings. By contrast, holidays such as Thanksgiving or Christmas, which put demands on you, can trigger high levels of stress. You may feel that commercialism detracts from the original meaning of the festival, or the expectation that you will spend time with your family puts too much pressure on you, either to travel great distances or to play host to an excess of feasting.

We may also be conditioned into taking on too many commitments, whether at work or in our social lives: volunteering for too many committees, or taking on yet another fund-raising event. The worst point is when you feel guilty about saying "no" to demands on your time. Negotiation and compromise are the key to balancing your own needs as a couple against the pressures and demands of your work place and your family circle. Demonstrate your willingness to be flexible and your commitment to work-place deadlines, but be sure you communicate the high value you place on your need for privacy and time off. With family, discuss your commitments and do your best to modify their expectations. Suggest that you spread your visits throughout the year, remembering birthdays and important anniversaries, as well as less formal engagements.

Negative stress has a nasty habit of creeping up on you. One of the key indicators is that something that you found stimulating a few weeks or months ago now seems like a chore, or even a threat. Symptoms of negative stress may also be physical: a dry or constricted throat, a tightness in the chest, or a nagging pain in the stomach. Worse still are sleeping problems, constant tiredness coupled with being unable to "switch off" on weekends, and loss of concentration.

The impact of many stress factors can be reduced by simple relaxation, visualization, and breathing techniques. Even during a busy working day, a couple of minutes spent easing your neck

Time to relax

Try this simple technique whenever you feel stressed. Note your breathing, and if it is rapid, return to normal, regular breaths. Slow down your breathing a little more, inhale slowly and smoothly, and breathe out through your mouth. Think about blowing out the candles on your birthday cake. Continue this slow phase for a few moments, then return to regular, steady breathing in your own time.

and shoulders, or taking a few deep breaths in the fresh air, can help. Contrary to some people's belief, smoking does not relieve your stress but will add to it.

High-quality nutrition is of the greatest importance: during times of stress the body uses up its store of minerals and requires higher levels of vitamins than usual. Make sure your nutrition levels are good, and take advice on extra supplements to boost your immune system.

Simple relaxation

- Give yourself permission to relax: set aside some time for yourself.
- Sit or lie comfortably in a quiet spot and close your eyes.
- Listen to the sound of your breathing for a moment or two. Let your thoughts come and go; don't give them attention.
- Now, count your in and out breaths. Breathe in…breathe out and count "one," breathe in…breathe out and count "two," up to ten.
- Repeat counting up to ten as many times as you want.
- When you are ready, gently open your eyes and give yourself time to "come to," before getting on with your day.

Make sense of the grieving process

From time to time, life presents us with shocks for which we are not prepared. The death of a loved one, particularly a close family member, is one example. Sometimes, even when we are prepared for the inevitable loss of a parent or grandparent, the moment of passing seems unbearable. Miscarriage can be equally devastating. The promise of future life seems crushed before you and your child have had a chance to enjoy it.

Returning to an emotional balance appears impossible, yet it is an important goal, for you and your family. It is essential to take time out at times of sudden shock and distress so you can allow the release of pain or grief to follow its own course. Sadness is a physiological process: our bodies respond to the natural ebbing and flowing of energy at these times. Traditionally, deep mourning lasted up to a year, when mourners would live a life of retreat from social pressures before gradually beginning to return to their normal routines. Scientists and the study of psycho-neuro-immunology have shown that the body takes this time to recover and restore the immune system and psychological balance.

Medical warning
If your stress symptoms continue, see your physician to check for underlying medical conditions. Take your physician's advice on relaxation techniques if you suffer from a heart condition, high blood pressure, or epilepsy.

There are known links between stress caused by the recent death of a close family member and reduction in sperm quality. Men experiencing such stress can suffer a temporary decline, but with time the body recovers its former fertility levels. Other strong emotions, such as feelings of guilt, can also block fertility. Discuss these issues in confidence with your clinician, counselor, or complementary therapist.

Stress disrupts the endocrine system—the system that sends hormonal signals to different parts of the bodies. These signals have a direct effect on fertility. They also upset our metabolism, and affect our appetite and sensations of taste. Many factors, such as our inner makeup, attitudes, and beliefs, play a part in the way we perceive stress, including the type, magnitude, and duration of the stress.

Counter the stress of subfertility

Even the decision to become future parents may be stressful to some couples. Many find medical investigations and tests invasive and threatening. Unrealistic expectations, such as expecting instant success, will put undue pressure on you both.

Concerns related to planning conception can have a negative impact on your fertility. "Firefighting" tactics, such as demanding daily sex in the hope of conceiving, are self-defeating and create avoidable tensions. Good timing is a far more effective route to conception—and needn't reduce spontaneity either! Sexual problems are also a cause of reduced fertility, and it is vitally important to address these sensitively and with professional support.

Your motivation and support for each other are key factors and are sometimes more important than medical details. There are well-documented cases of spontaneous fertility—even among supposedly infertile couples—which continue to puzzle doctors and experts. A change of pace, fewer responsibilities, a move to parttime employment or to a quieter part of the country, may all have the effect of relaxing you and triggering successful conception.

Stress will not, in itself, keep you from conceiving or having a healthy baby—although it may slow down the time you take to conceive. By reducing stress levels during your countdown to conception, you will have more time to enjoy your new lifestyle.

Analyze your stress factors

Take a piece of paper and write down the major stress factors in your life at present. Write against each one whether you feel that whatever is causing the stress is within your control or outside your control.

Are these stress factors having an adverse effect on your social standing—with your friends, in the work place or within your family? Finally consider how long the stress has been going on—less than three months, three to six months, up to one year, or more than one year?

The next step is to put the stress factors aside for a moment and do one of the simple relaxation techniques described on pages 62–63.

Now, think about what actions you can take to reduce stress. Do you feel under pressure from your family—or is it mainly work-related?

Do you need to attend a time-management or assertiveness training course? Should you talk to your employers about your workload or difficult staff relationships? Do you need to spend time with a professional counselor or enroll in yoga or relaxation classes? Whatever is best for you, integrate your personal stress management program into the countdown for conception (see pages 116–125).

Give yourself the time and space to let go of your stress. Chapter 4 includes some relaxation, exercise, and complementary therapy ideas to help you unwind and enjoy your life.

Stress factor	PSYCHOLOGICAL STRESS		SOCIAL STRESS AFFECTING RELATIONSHIPS			MAGNITUDE OF STRESS				DURATION OF STRESS				ACTION PLAN
	Within my control	*Outside my control*	*Friends*	*Work place*	*Family*	*Most stressful*	*Very stressful*	*Fairly stressful*	*Mildly stressful*	*Less than 3 months*	*3–6 months*	*6–12 months*	*Over 1 year*	*Including medical checkup exercise, work place training, counseling, aromatherapy*
Example	X		X						X	X				Exercise

Start an exercise routine

Regular exercise can benefit your health by improving your immune system, boosting your circulation, raising your energy levels, and stretching your muscles. The best type of exercise for you will depend upon your current state of health and vitality, so take advice from your physician. You should be able to do your chosen exercise easily, regularly, and safely. It is important not to overdo your exercise—overtraining can have the opposite effect and reduce your immune system at a time when you need to improve your resistance to infection. If you choose something you enjoy, you will be more likely to keep up the regime.

Exercise that combines relaxation with stretching, such as t'ai chi and yoga, will help reduce your stress levels, as well as building you up physically. Alternately, you may want to improve your lung capacity and stamina, so cycling, swimming, or aerobics might be best. Dancing together is a lighthearted way of burning off calories, as well as toning your muscles: choose your favorite music and enjoy yourselves!

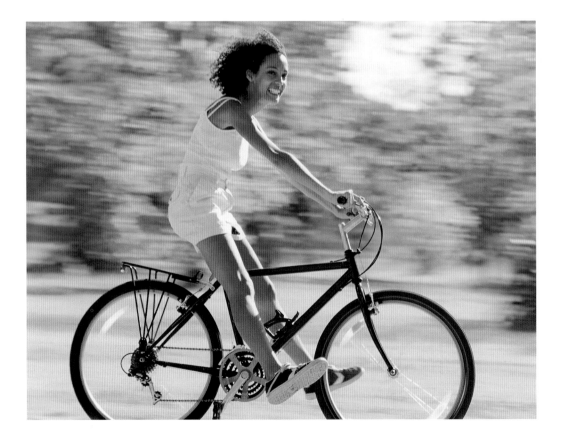

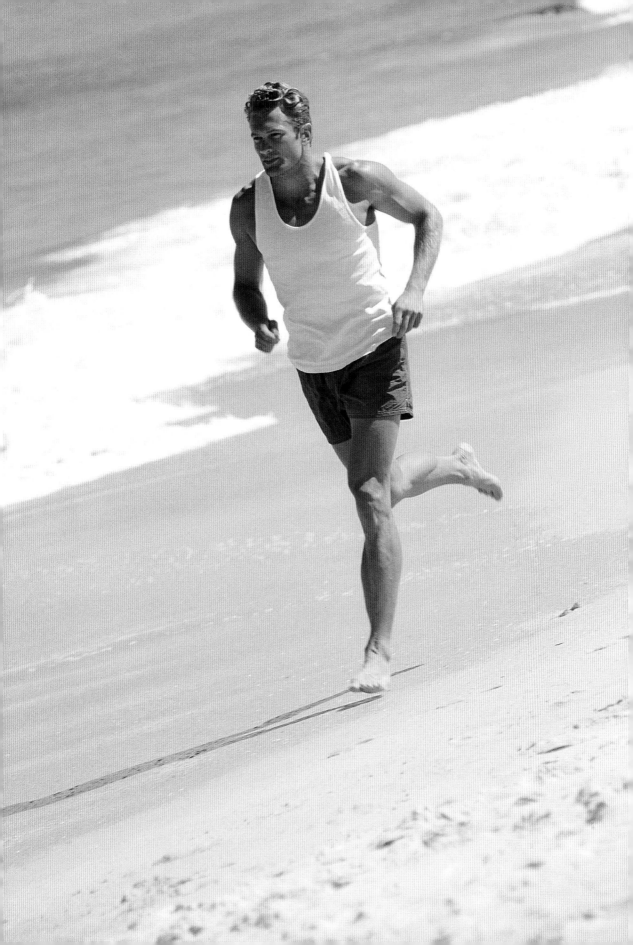

Chapter three

Fertility awareness

A practical understanding of fertility awareness is important for a healthy conception and helps you to work in harmony with your personal cycles. This section looks at male and female reproductive systems and the factors that affect your fertility.

Fertility is a sensitive issue. Men are still getting used to the fact that they have a fertility cycle and that their health level, as well as their partner's, is vital in achieving a successful, healthy conception. Don't let scare stories about sperm counts worry you—your clinician can regularly monitor your sperm, and only one strong, healthy sperm is needed to fertilize an egg. You can both test your fertility levels regularly—in some cases using convenient home-testing techniques.

Personal and sexual health can also be a sensitive matter. There are many conditions that affect fertility but do not present symptoms. Known as "subclinical" conditions, they are responsible for many previously unexplained fertility factors. Checking for preexisting infections will improve your wellbeing and fertility. Knowing about medications that affect fertility levels allows you to discuss options with your clinician.

Fertility awareness is knowledge to be shared. Few fertility counselors or clinicians will now meet one partner alone because interacting factors may be responsible for your failure to conceive. Most importantly, such consultations are a way of offering you support at a time when you both need it. Use this book as a backup to any medical advice you receive and as a checklist for the questions you may want to ask. Your clinician will confirm whether a particular issue is relevant to you and will offer specific treatment options, where necessary.

This section contains an overview of how male and female reproductive systems work. It describes the importance of luteinizing hormone (LH) testing, ways of charting your primary fertility signs, and the "symptothermal" method of fertility awareness for women—using your early morning or "basal body" temperature together with other key signals to predict ovulation. It shows you how to keep a chart to help you maximize your chances of conception—particularly

Understanding each other is an important part of preparing for conception. The better informed you are about physical and emotional issues, the easier it will be to deal with any worries or problems that do arise.

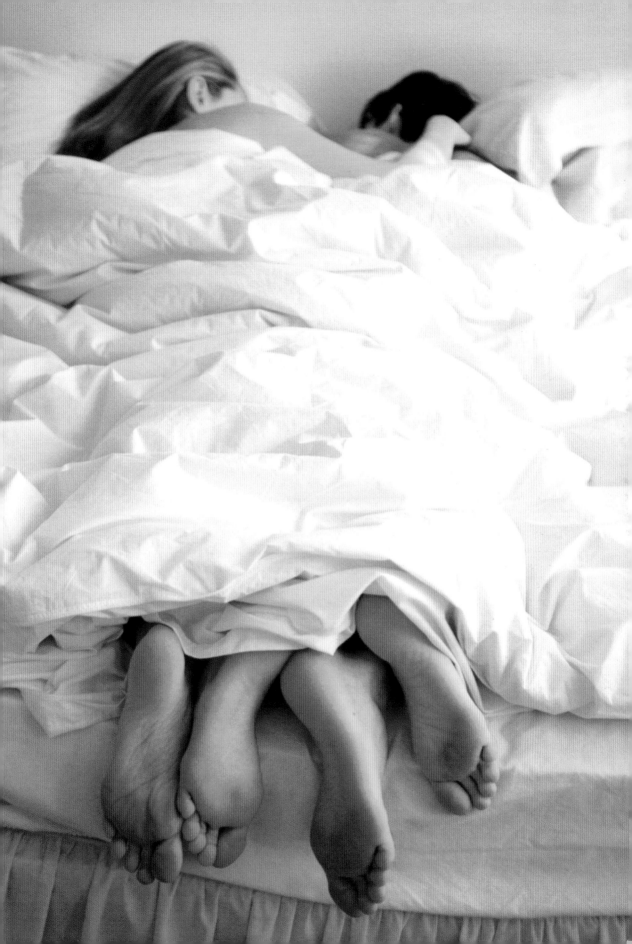

important if you have recently suffered a miscarriage or experienced a long phase of infertility. Using the countdown to conception, you can chart your fertility cycle, generate new sperm in tiptop condition, and reach optimum health and fitness in as little as three months.

Restoring the balance

A healthy woman's ovulatory cycle should be about 28 days, and a mature egg (ovum) is normally released around the mid-point of this cycle. The opportunity for fertilization to take place lasts about three to five days, and the egg needs a fertile environment in which to survive and fuse with the sperm. If the egg is not

Conception: the key factors

Three key factors interact to create a healthy conception.

One: Male

The quality of your sperm. It needs to be strong, mobile, and well formed. Healthy sperm are developed by good diet, gentle exercise, and avoiding harmful toxins.

Two: Female

The quality of your eggs and their ability to travel along your fallopian tubes. Absence of infection and blockages will improve your chances of conception and a healthy pregnancy.

Three: Both

The compatibility of your sperm and vaginal fluids, neither of which should contain auto-antibodies. The vaginal fluid is most receptive when it is alkaline and can encourage sperm motility. A postcoital test can identify any problems, which can then be resolved.

The common factor that will boost your sperm, eggs, fallopian tubes, and fluids is nutrition: the B-complex vitamins, vitamin C, and zinc all help.

In cases of infections or blockages, antibiotic treatment may be necessary. Complementary treatments, such as homeopathy or acupuncture, can also help trigger your self-healing mechanisms (see Chapter 4 for more details).

fertilized, it, and the lining of the womb, break down
and the monthly menstruation, or period, takes place.

The 28-day cycle is an important marker for menstrual health,
although the exact timing varies from woman to woman and
from month to month. External factors, such as stress, dieting,
or medication, can upset the normal delicate balance, which
must be corrected before conception can be successful. This
is why it is important to chart your own ovulatory cycles and
understand your personal patterns. Knowing when you ovulate
also reduces the stress of continuously trying to conceive and
the pressures this can cause: you can target your lovemaking
and set aside special times to be together.

Take time to boost your fertility—rushing into conception
will not give your child the best start in life. Men create sperm
in batches on a continuous basis, with a typical development
time of about 90 days (roughly three months). In that time, they
can benefit from a high-quality diet and a healthy lifestyle which
will improve sperm quality. The sperm carry half of the genetic
makeup of the future child and need to be able to survive and
swim up to the egg during the fertile phase.

Men can improve their sperm count and quality in just the
same way as building muscle tone. Reduce stress, improve
your nutritional levels and overall health, and your sperm
will automatically increase in strength and abundance. For
those with preexisting medical conditions, problems with
toxic overload, or a low sperm count, regaining fertility may
take longer, once the underlying factors have been resolved
and appropriate action taken.

Countdown to conception

Use the "Countdown to conception" plan (Chapter 5)
to prepare for a healthy conception and look at the lifestyle
changes suggested in Chapter 2. Give yourselves at least three
months to chart your ovulatory cycle and improve your sperm
quality; allow six months if you have a history of miscarriage
or low sperm count, and longer if you have preexisting
medical conditions or a history of infertility.

When you are both ready, you can plan your conception with
the confidence that comes from understanding your natural
cycles. The countdown to conception is not rushed: it gives you
both time to discover how your bodies really work. In this way
conception is more likely, and you will develop sensitivity and
a greater appreciation of each other. You can share your
knowledge and harmonize your countdown to conception.

Male fertility

Nature is abundant without being wasteful and the potential exists for men to be fertile well into old age. In each ejaculation millions of sperm are released into a woman's body, only one of which needs to be successful. A man's sperm needs to be strong and well shaped, as well as energetic and mobile. It needs to survive for three to five days as it impregnates the fertile egg.

Men experience their most important physical changes at puberty, and this transitional phase has major implications for the rest of their reproductive life. These changes create what are known as the "primary" and "secondary" sexual characteristics. Men then continue to develop sperm throughout their adult life —unless interrupted by stress or illness—although typically a decline in quality begins at around age 50.

The testes

The testes produce sperm and secrete male sex hormones, known as androgens. The best-known androgen is testosterone, which is responsible for the development of secondary sexual characteristics: facial and body hair, deepening of the voice, and muscle and bone development.

The testes are held in a soft muscular pouch called the scrotum. This needs to be outside the body because the testes require a temperature a degree or two below normal body temperature. The muscles can contract to move the scrotum closer to the body when cold and can give off heat if necessary. This need for a cool environment explains the advice often given to men who want to increase their fertility level, such as not to wear over-tight clothes, reduce time spent in cramped driving conditions, and take cool baths to improve sperm quality.

Each testis is divided into about 300 areas, all containing seminiferous tubules. These are tubes lined with rapidly dividing cells that produce the sperm. The tubules form ducts, or passages, for the sperm to travel down.

The male reproductive system is designed to produce and store sperm on a continuous basis and to make sure they reach the female's egg in tiptop condition.

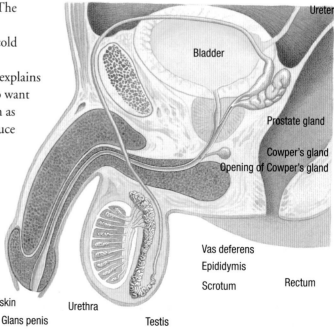

Seminal vesicle

Ureter

Bladder

Prostate gland

Cowper's gland

Opening of Cowper's gland

Vas deferens

Epididymis

Scrotum

Rectum

Foreskin

Urethra

Glans penis

Testis

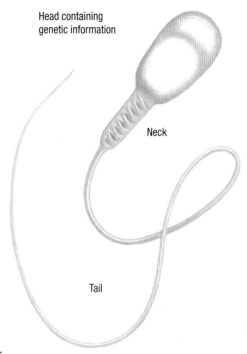

Head containing
genetic information

Neck

Tail

*Propelled by its whiplike tail, the
sperm travels to penetrate the egg
and achieve fertilization.*

Each of these passages lead to an epididymis, where the sperm
is stored while it matures. The epididymis in turn leads to the
muscular sperm ducts, called the vas deferens. These ducts
open into the urethra—the tube running from the bladder
through the length of the penis to the outside. A complex
network of circular muscle at the base of the bladder prevents
urine from entering the urethra at the same time as the
sperm. The penis shaft itself is made from soft tissue, which
fills with blood when the man is aroused, enabling sexual
intercourse to take place.

Sperm

Sperm is constantly produced in the testes. A healthy man
can produce 50,000 sperm a minute, which is an incredible
72 million every day. These sperm travel to the epididymis
where they mature over a 72-day period, then break down
and are absorbed back into the system if they are not ejaculated.

Each tiny sperm is made up of three parts, which are visible
under a microscope:

- The head contains the chromosomes and genetic information
  that are the male contribution to the child's heredity.
- The neck is a system of nerves that nourish the sperm,
  creating an energy supply and aiding movement.
- The tail is the "motor," which propels the sperm forward
  by lashing energetically from side to side, using stored
  glucose as its "fuel."

It is important that sperm are well shaped and include these
characteristics so that they can reach and penetrate the egg.
The term "motility" describes the capacity of a sperm to move
and its strength of movement: it is an important characteristic.

The sperm is forced out through the urethra by rhythmic
contractions of the epididymis, sperm ducts, and other muscles,
giving enough thrust for the sperm to have the best chance of
fusion with the egg.

Seminal fluid

Sperm alone is not enough. For it to make the journey
successfully and fuse with an egg, sperm must be nourished
by a rich fluid. The seminal fluid is protective, energizing,
and lubricating, and is also composed of three parts.

Contents of seminal fluid

➥ An alkaline fluid,
produced by two seminal
vesicles, or pouches, which
protects the sperm from
any acidity in the female
vaginal fluid.
➥ A fluid containing
glucose, released by the
prostate gland, which
enables the sperm to move
rapidly and sustain energy.
➥ A preejaculatory fluid,
produced by the Cowper's
glands at the end of the
urethra, which acts as a
lubricant along the path
taken by the ejaculate.

Female fertility

Because of a precisely synchronized process, triggered by the release of the hormones estrogen and progesterone, several changes take place in a woman's body during the course of the menstrual cycle:

- A surge of luteinizing hormone (LH) announces forthcoming ovulation.
- Temperature changes, peaking at ovulation.
- A mature egg is released.
- Fluids that help to carry the sperm to the egg increase.
- The cervix changes shape, height, opening, and angle.

Your body will give you useful clues as to when this is happening so you can learn to recognize and chart your fertile phases. You can also buy simple home-testing kits to check your hormone levels and anticipate ovulation.

Learning your body language

Eggs are stored in a woman's body from birth, but from adolescence onward, they develop from immature "oocytes" into mature eggs as they are needed. Women store their eggs within the ovaries and usually just one is released each month. This is known as ovulation. The egg then travels down the fallopian tube and into the womb, where it can be fertilized by a single sperm. If you know when you ovulate, you can time your lovemaking more precisely and improve your chances of conception and pregnancy.

In some circumstances, more than one egg may be released in a cycle—this is the process that is encouraged in assisted fertility (see pages 126–129). Conversely, it is not unusual for women not to release an egg; no two months are exactly the same and no two women are the same. Because of this, it is important to understand your particular cycle.

Charting your fertility signs

Photocopy and enlarge the chart on page 131 and follow the guidelines for recording your temperature. This is known as the symptothermal method of fertility awareness. You may be shy at first about focusing on your body this way and discussing your fertility signals with your partner, but it's important to get to know your body better. Taking notes and recording temperatures will soon become routine.

Failure to conceive
Sometimes, failure to conceive may be due to a simple factor, such as the woman's fluid being too acidic to receive the sperm. Your clinician may advise a bicarbonate of soda douche, which makes the fluid more alkaline and solves the problem.

Plotting a chart means you can:

- Identify the length of your average cycle.
- Establish whether or not you are ovulating and, if not, to take action to help restore ovulation.
- Link physical symptoms with particular phases in your cycle.
- Improve unwanted symptoms caused by stress or poor diet.
- Help your clinician identify a particular cause if you are having problems conceiving.
- Anticipate your most fertile phase, when you are ready to conceive.

Factors to take into account

Any one of these may affect or stop your menstrual cycle:

- Your age: the length of your menstrual cycle decreases from a typical 29 days at about age 20, to nearly 27 days at age 40.
- Your weight: whether you are underweight or overweight, coming back to an appropriate average will improve your personal wellbeing and enhance your fertility levels.
- Anxiety and stress.
- Your nutritional status, which needs to be good for a healthy conception and pregnancy.
- Alcohol, medication, or recreational drugs.
- Environmental hazards, such as chemicals, pesticides, and household products (see Chapter 2).

Temperature: a primary fertility signal

In addition to a copy of the chart, you will need a basal body thermometer to measure your daily temperature. Because this records body temperature only within a narrow range, the tube of mercury is very thin and is held under magnified glass. It takes time to learn how to read a basal body thermometer— there is a knack to it! Check your readings a few times until you are sure you understand the thermometer correctly.

When you are ready, set aside a little time each morning to take your temperature and note it down on your chart. Do this before you get up to go to the bathroom or have your first morning drink. Soon a regular pattern should emerge. Don't expect your chart always to remain the same. Most women have

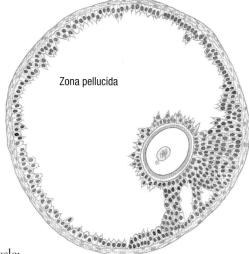

Zona pellucida

Nucleus

This mature egg has been released from the ovary and is ready to be fertilized. The complex mix of hormones shifts, and calcium levels rise significantly. The successful sperm binds with the zona pellucida. It moves through this shell toward the oocyte, where it fuses and creates a two-cell "conceptus"—the start of a rapidly growing fetus.

three distinct points of change in their overall cycle, and your temperature can rise and fall even within these.

1 Body temperature is low before ovulation
Early morning temperature is normally a little below the more familiar figure of 98.6°F and it is slightly lower during the first half of the cycle than the second. This difference may be only a fraction of a degree, which is why fertility thermometers have expanded scales, showing just a few degrees of temperature.

2 Your temperature at ovulation dips and then peaks
This is the moment when the egg is released and your fertile phase begins. If intercourse takes place within 24 hours, it offers the best opportunity for successful conception.

3 Your temperature rises a little and stays high until menstruation
Your temperature will be a little above the level recorded in the first half of your cycle and will stay around this level until your period begins.

The countdown to conception recommends that you keep a chart for at least three months to familiarize yourself with your cycle. Your body temperature can be affected by factors such as stress, late nights, infection, or even alcohol drunk the night before. Follow the countdown to conception regime and aim to eliminate such factors before you try to conceive.

If you find that you are not ovulating, or that there are marked differences between each monthly cycle, seek medical advice or talk to your fertility adviser.

Identifying your LH surge

LH stands for "luteinizing hormone," a special hormone that is released by the body approximately 24–36 hours before ovulation. It is linked to the moment when your egg is released from an ovary and begins to travel down a fallopian tube to your womb. The hormone is passed out of the body in urine and can be easily tested for at home.

If you want to check if you are ovulating when you begin your countdown plan, you can purchase a home-testing kit to identify your LH surge. Later in your countdown, when you have gotten to know your cycle, you can pinpoint the time of ovulation more precisely using this type of test.

The LH test is similar in approach to home pregnancy tests, but it is searching for a different hormone in your urine. Kits

Vaginal fluids
Getting to know your own body's signs and signals depends on careful observation. Your clinician or a nurse can show you how to identify and record signs that can improve your chances of conception.

usually come with several testing sticks, which means that, as long as you know your typical cycle length, you can check every day for a few days. The instructions supplied with the testing kits show you how to figure out how and when to start. Results will appear in around five minutes.

It is important to take the test at about the same time each day, but you can choose the time that suits you. An LH surge is not a guarantee of ovulation, and it can occasionally show a "false positive" result, particularly if you are already pregnant or are approaching menopause. Some drugs given to assist conception may also confuse the result, and you should check with your clinician as to whether an LH test would be suitable.

If your cycle varies from month to month by more than three days, you may find it helpful to chart your basal body temperature carefully and time the use of the LH surge test in combination with your temperature changes.

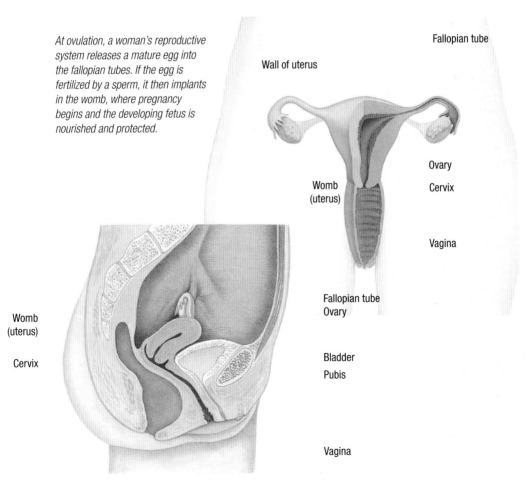

At ovulation, a woman's reproductive system releases a mature egg into the fallopian tubes. If the egg is fertilized by a sperm, it then implants in the womb, where pregnancy begins and the developing fetus is nourished and protected.

Fallopian tube

Wall of uterus

Womb (uterus)

Ovary

Cervix

Vagina

Fallopian tube
Ovary

Bladder
Pubis

Womb (uterus)

Cervix

Vagina

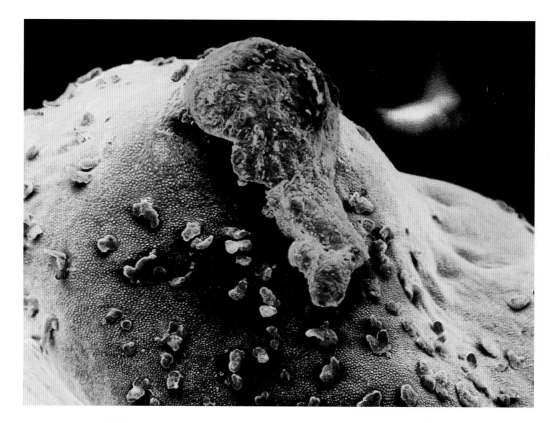

Background body signals

The combination of basal body temperature and LH surge testing will give you a firm indication as to when you are ovulating and the best time to try to conceive. In addition to this information, your body may be giving you other signals, alerting you to your fertile cycle.

Symptoms such as tenderness or bloated feelings are associated with fertility. These are all secondary signs, not experienced by all women. Your secondary signals will help confirm your fertile phase and can be charted alongside your temperature and LH surge. You may experience:

- **Aches and pains:** a sharp pain at ovulation on one side of the groin or the other. This happens as the egg is released into your fallopian tube and may turn into a dull ache for up to a day or so.
- **Spotting:** small spots of blood, known as mid-cycle bleeding.
- **Tingling:** a sense of breast "tingling" or tenderness after ovulation, as estrogens are released into your system.
- **Bowel pressure:** a sense of "pressure" in the rectum, or tension

This highly magnified picture shows the surface of a woman's ovary at the time of ovulation. Beneath the swollen surface at the top is an egg, ready to be released into the fallopian tube. Your full complement of eggs is stored in your ovaries from birth. They grow and mature in a regular cycle from puberty until menopause.

during bowel movements, which may be associated with painful hemorrhoids.

Vaginal fluids

Women continually create lubricating fluid in the cervix which flows into the vagina. At different points in the cycle, in harmony with the infertile and fertile phases, this changes from a scant, creamy discharge to a clear slippery fluid. Some women experience abundant "egg-white" type fluid indicating a peak fertility day.

- **Infertile:** You will be most "dry" at the stage before ovulation, when your cervix is sealed by a sticky liquid, known as mucus. The mucus is densely structured to block attempts by the sperm to enter. Also, the vaginal passage is acidic, preventing the sperm from flourishing.
- **Fertile:** As your egg ripens, the vaginal fluid becomes increasingly damp and "stretchy" until it becomes abundant, clear, and slippery. At this point your egg is ripe, and the vaginal fluid is a perfect alkaline medium for receiving and nurturing sperm.

Observation of these changes will help you recognize your fertile phase. Avoid the use of spermicidal creams or lubricating gels in the time before you are planning to conceive, especially those containing an ingredient called nonoxynol 9. This creates an acid environment that kills sperm and may encourage cystitis.

Cervix positions
◗ Infertile phase: the cervix falls; fluid is thick and mucuslike
◗ Fertile phase: the cervix rises; fluid is clear, slippery, and abundant.

Cervical position

The cervix is normally closed and sealed with the mucus plug, but during the cycle it changes in four ways: shape, height, opening, and angle. During your fertile phase, as estrogen levels rise, your cervix will move into a high position, directly in line with your vaginal opening.

The cervix has a cylindrical shape, about 1 inch in diameter, with a small dimple (known as the "os") in the middle. It is this dimple that opens up each month to receive fertile sperm into the uterus. If you have previously had a baby, the dimple may never be totally closed.

Knowing your cervical position is not a firm indicator of fertility, since different hormones are required to release an egg from the ovary, and the cervix may rise and fall without an egg being released. However, your family-planning nurse or fertility clinician may wish to check your cervix and may recommend home examination. They can show you how to check its position in the privacy of your home.

The female fertility cycle

Your fertility changes over a regular cycle, which may last from 24 to 32 days. Record alterations in the four key signs to check your peak fertility time: base body temperature, background body signals, vaginal fluids, and cervix position. It may take a little practice to learn how to recognize these changes, but you

The female fertility cycle

Phase	Duration	Base body temperature
Menstruation phase (period)	First day of menstruation is considered day one of your cycle.	Temperature drops back.
Preovulation or "follicular" phase	Pre-ovulation phase lasts 10-14 days.	Temperature in the first half of cycle is generally a point or two lower than in second half.
Ovulation phase LH surge Peak fertility days	Ovulation usually occurs in the middle of the cycle, between day 12 and day 16. This may vary from month to month.	Temperature drops and then rises.
Still in fertile phase Becoming less fertile toward period	Post-ovulation or "luteal" phase lasts 12–15 days.	Temperature generally stays a point or two higher than in your preovulation phase.
Menstruation phase (period)	Whole cycle lasts 24–32 days.	Temperature drops back.

will soon get used to it, and your physician can show you how to check your cervix. Don't worry if you do not have all the background body signals—just note the ones you do experience. Photocopy the chart on page 131 and use it to record your cycle changes and help you to pinpoint your fertile time.

Background signals	Vaginal fluid signals	Cervix changes
Clinician may ask you to note the volume of blood loss, color, and degree of clotting.		
Sexual desire may be low.	**Feeling:** moist or damp. **Color:** white, cloudy, or opaque. **Amount:** sparse or abundant. **Texture:** creamy, crumbly, or elastic.	**Position:** low—within easy reach and tilted away from vaginal opening. **Shape:** firm, long, and cone shaped. **Texture:** dry, gritty surface. **Dimple:** closed.
Ovulation pain. Mid-cycle "spotting" or bleeding. Increased sex drive.	**Feeling:** wet. **Color:** transparent. **Amount:** abundant. **Texture:** similar to egg white.	**Position:** high. **Dimple:** wide enough to admit finger.
Heaviness of breasts. Water retention. Bowel pressure.	**Feeling:** wet—well lubricated. **Color:** cloudy, clear, or transparent. **Amount:** abundant. **Texture:** slippery, stretchy, or like egg white.	**Position:** higher—harder to reach and tilted toward vaginal opening. **Shape:** soft and flabby. **Texture:** wet—covered in fluid. **Dimple:** open.

Understanding subfertility

Although one egg requires only one sperm, the quality of both
is crucial. A healthy conception requires mature sperm, which
are strong and energetic, and have been well nourished during
their creation, maturing, and ejaculation phases. The sperm
need to be able to fertilize an egg that is also mature and strong
enough to survive the rigors of rapid cell division and growth.
A healthy sperm that successfully meets and fuses with a mature
egg creates a lasting message of vitality for your future child.

It sounds so simple, yet only 50 percent of couples conceive
during their first three months of trying. This rises to about
70 percent within six months, but some couples may not
manage to conceive within their first year. This is perfectly
normal, yet the waiting can become stressful if you are eager
to start a family. For older couples, the chances are that
conception will take six months or longer.

You may feel under greater stress when your physician uses
terms such as "subfertile" or "infertility." These are clinical
definitions, which sound threatening and may be used by
different clinicians to mean different things! These are the
common terms used to describe fertility:

- **Subfertile** indicates a couple who have not conceived within
  12 months. You may not be offered medical tests within this
  time, and you may be advised to "go away and keep trying."
  However, you can improve your fertility levels, even without
  medical assistance (see Chapter 2 Boosting your fertility and
  Chapter 5 Countdown to conception).
- **Infertility** is often defined as the inability to conceive within
  24 months. Seek medical help after 12 months if you have
  not already done so.
- **Primary infertility** means that a couple have not yet
  succeeded in conceiving a child.
- **Secondary infertility** means that a couple may have
  succeeded on one or more occasions in the past but are
  having difficulty now.
- **Sterility** means that conception is physically ruled out—a
  situation which affects only 1 percent of couples.
- **Infertility of unexplained origin** means that in theory
  no particular problems have been detected, but in practice
  conception has not yet happened. There is, typically, a need
  for detailed and careful testing for couples in this situation
  and this does take time.

If you have been trying for more than a year, it is important to have a medical checkup and a number of fertility tests. You can find out whether, for example, you have a low sperm count or ovulate rarely. You can then take the specific actions necessary to boost your fertility and perhaps target your lovemaking around peak fertility times.

Sexual problems: mind over matter?

One of the main causes of failure to conceive, especially of infertility of unknown origin, are the psychological factors linked to sex. If these are addressed at an early stage, you may avoid the need for fertility tests and medical treatment completely. Women are known to react to infertility through increased thoughts and concerns regarding conception. This can lead to repetitive or "obsessive" behavior, which can be stressful for both partners.

The worry of subfertility can be a cause of partnership stresses which, in turn, may trigger a number of sexual problems, such as impotence, premature ejaculation, or vaginal spasm. On the other hand, these disorders may be the underlying reason for subfertility. They are not uncommon problems, particularly when one of you is unwell or under work or social pressure. It's like a vicious circle, isn't it?

Men's sense of self, their sexuality, and the wish to conceive can also create sexual problems. Impotence can be caused by a variety of problems, such as fatigue, stress, and illness. Certain drugs, toxins, additives, and neurological problems caused by spinal injuries or diseases can also be a cause.

The important thing is to break this cycle of stress and take the pressure off. Lovemaking is meant to be a pleasure—a balance between recreation and procreation. For fertility, our bodies work best when both aspects are in harmony. If you seek counseling or other help, the first advice will often be to relax and focus on other aspects of your lovemaking, such as sharing affection through massage or extended foreplay. Chapter 4 suggests a range of holistic activities to relax your bodies and improve your wellbeing, and these will also help to reduce any sexual tensions.

Despite the open society we now live in and the wide selection of books, magazines, and other explicit material, infertility can still be caused by non-consummation or "defective coital technique." The physical location of a woman's cervix, for

A different approach
Charles Buck practices traditional Chinese acupuncture and herbal medicine. His success with fertility problems gives him confidence that these treatments are appropriate for infertility, even where IVF has failed.

Claire, a midwife in her early forties, had been married for a couple of years to Simon, and they desperately wanted to have a child before time ran out. Investigations showed that Claire was fine, but Simon had both low sperm counts and low motility.

The typical treatment is a classic Chinese herbal prescription for 16 weeks, but Claire was in a big hurry. She arranged a re-test for Simon after only two weeks. Simon's count and motility had almost doubled, and Claire became pregnant during that cycle.

example, may simply require a different position when making love in order to assist the sperm toward the egg.

It cannot be said often enough: "size doesn't matter!"—either of the penis or testes. What is important is the *quality* of the sperm and egg. If you still have concerns about your size or shape, ask for a medical checkup or for professional counseling. Do not allow anxiety about your physique to create a barrier to fertility—or your everyday happiness. Help is now readily available to allow couples to cope with this and many other problems and improve their chances of conception.

Fertility testing

If your lovemaking is usually without problems and you have been trying to conceive for more than three months, you may wish to ask your clinician for a medical checkup and fertility tests. The typical causes of subfertility, described in more detail below, are:

- Tubal damage: blocked sperm ducts or fallopian tubes.
- Problems associated with ovulation, including endometriosis.
- Problems associated with sperm.

The likelihood of conception will vary, depending on the severity of the problem and the length of time you have had the particular condition. There is a series of straightforward tests, available for both partners, which can identify the causes and help your clinician offer solutions. You can also do a great deal to improve your fertility levels and overall wellbeing using the advice in this book.

Autoimmune responses

In certain circumstances our own bodies can trigger illnesses known as autoimmune responses, which may affect fertility. They occur, for example, when sperm cells cross natural barriers, invade other cell types, and trigger the body's immune system—as if a hostile substance has entered the body.

This can lead to inflammation of the testis, commonly associated with subfertility. "Clumping" describes a situation when auto-antibodies deactivate the sperm, causing them to "clump" together and lose their motility.

Cervical mucus can stimulate an immune response which prevents sperm from penetrating—again, responding to it as a "hostile" substance. Bacteria present in the ejaculate may also affect the ability of sperm to penetrate the cervical mucus,

Tests: what to expect from your clinician

In addition to taking a complete medical history from you both, your clinician will want you to have a thorough medical examination, possibly using ultrasound, and a check for infections and inflammations. Here are some specific investigations you may be recommended to undergo:

Condition	What to expect in tests
Endometriosis Tests carried out by a gynecologist	A "laparoscope," a small instrument like a special camera with a light attached, is used to look initially at the pelvic area of the body. A small incision is made, near the navel, to insert the laparoscope under anesthetic.
Tubal damage Tests usually carried out by a gynecologist for women and an andrologist for men	Physical examination, which may include ultrasound. Full medical history taken. Hormone levels checked—typically at different times of the month.
Ovulation problems carried out by your physician or gynecologist	Physical examination plus: ultrasound to check ovaries and uterus; cervical smear to check cervix; blood tests to check hormone levels.
Sperm problems Tests carried out by your physician or fertility specialist	Physical examination plus: sperm test to check for number, shape, and motility; blood tests to check hormone levels. Ask about the availability of home-testing equipment.
Sperm/mucus compatibility Tests carried out by your physician or fertility specialist	Postcoital test to check for antibodies. Ask about the availability of home testing.
Hormone sampling Tests carried out by your preconceptional care clinician	Non-invasive techniques, such as sampling of saliva to check estrogen and progesterone levels.

without any signs or symptoms to indicate a problem. A special postcoital test can check whether your sperm and cervical mucus are compatible, and other tests are available to check for the presence of anerobic bacteria.

Once detected, steps can be taken to improve the situation. These may be as straightforward as recommending simple vitamin C or E, or zinc and other supplements, but some couples may need more specialized treatment.

Endometriosis

The endometrium is an inner layer of the wall of the womb (uterus), which changes in structure and thickness during the menstrual cycle. These changes allow the wall to become receptive to the fertilized egg for a very brief time. If an egg is not fertilized or implanted into the endometrium, the result is the monthly bleeding, or period.

In endometriosis, this endometrial tissue develops outside the womb. It is normal tissue and goes through the same preparation and shedding cycle as its counterpart in the womb, but for some reason, it grows in the wrong places. This causes bleeding, which can lead to cysts forming on the ovary as well as scar tissue where the endometrial tissue contacts other organs such as intestines. The cyclical changes in these endometrial areas lead to pain and inflammation around the time of the menstrual period and eventual scars that can cause all manner of problems, including the blockage of the fallopian tubes, bowel problems, and pelvic pain.

The causes of endometriosis are not fully understood, but may be due to the following:

- Overproduction of estrogen.
- Genetic factors—endometriosis does run in families.
- Menstrual tissue flowing back into the fallopian tubes.
- Links between candidiasis and endometriosis if there is a history of vaginal thrush, overuse of antibiotics, and allergic symptoms.

Endometriosis need not prevent conception, although mild endometriosis is regularly diagnosed in women with fertility problems. Ironically, pregnancy may even alleviate symptoms and delay recurrence; endometriosis typically stops altogether after menopause.

Nutritional treatment, including herbal supplements, can help alleviate the symptoms of endometriosis and deal with underlying causes. In more severe cases, surgical techniques can help, including keyhole surgery.

Fertility problems caused by tubal damage

Blocked or twisted tubes or ducts can be a problem for either partner. Blockages can be caused by previous infections or allergic reactions. The typical treatment is to clear infections using antibiotics, followed up with supplements such as acidophilus and zinc. Tubal problems are more frequent in smokers and may be linked to vitamin C deficiency. Sufferers will be advised to stop smoking if they hope to conceive.

If obstructions have caused blockages for a long time— typically more than six years—the damage may not be reversible and assisted conception may be necessary. Sometimes, for example, fallopian tubes will have suffered severe physical damage from past pelvic inflammatory disease or endometriosis. In these cases, pregnancy may not be achieved through sexual intercourse, and you may be advised to try assisted pregnancy techniques. This is also true of men who have had a vasectomy and are now seeking a reversal. A reversal may or may not restore potency, and sperm may not be capable of fertilization.

In men, blockages in the tubes taking seminal fluid from the testicles may be caused by infections such as mumps. Another common problem is a twisting or dilation of veins, known as a varicocele, which can be successfully corrected by microsurgery, involving minimal anesthetic and a few days off work. This condition is normally identified and treated when the young man is between 10 and 18 years old.

Testicular cancer is becoming an increasing problem. Typically occurring between the ages of 19 and 34, it is the most common cancer in men. While testicular cancer can be successfully treated, it can leave men unable to conceive, and the stress of a diagnosis can have an effect, as well as the disease itself. The psychological impacts can be very high and may affect your intimate relationships. There are ways to help: pretreatment planning can allow for sperm to be collected and safely stored for later assisted fertility treatment.

Undescended testicles

Since the testes require a cooler environment than normal body temperature, they descend from within the body before birth or during the first couple of years of life. If this does not occur, either for hormonal or other reasons, problems with fertility can arise. Treatment is usually carried out before puberty and is generally successful. Rarely, adults can be affected, and homeopathy can help in these cases. Once treated, fertility levels and chances of conception should be normal.

Fertility problems associated with ovulation

The number of eggs stored by mature women is of much less importance than their quality and the presence of a regular ovulatory cycle. Ovulation has two key phases: the follicular (roughly the first twelve days of the cycle) and the luteal (the second half of the cycle after ovulation). The follicular phase is triggered by a hormone known as FSH (follicle-stimulating hormone) associated with the hormone estrogen, which is responsible for releasing a mature egg. The moment of ovulation is connected with the LH surge (described on pages 76–77). The luteal phase is also associated with progesterone, which is secreted in readiness for conception and possible pregnancy.

Difficulties with conception may be linked to either phase of the cycle. By determining the different hormone levels, your clinician can pinpoint the problem area. If you have recently stopped taking the pill, your body may take time to readjust and allow your own hormones to regain their natural rhythm. Hormonal imbalances, caused by illness, stress, or nutritional deficiencies, may affect your ovaries or the endometrium. The imbalance may affect ovulation, which might stop completely.

Infection and the resulting inflammation and scar tissue may be caused by pelvic inflammatory disease (PID), or by the use of an intrauterine device (IUD or "coil"), resulting in blockages or damage to the womb or fallopian tubes. PID is also associated with past venereal disease.

Ovaries can become enlarged and covered in pearl-white cysts, a condition known as polycystic ovaries. This may be linked to excessive levels of androgens (better known as male hormones) or the condition may be due to pituitary gland problems. The ovaries become unable to produce the hormones needed to ripen the follicle or develop the womb lining. The womb itself may be damaged by surgery, including post-childbirth, or by abortion, infection, or the growth of polyps or precancerous cells. Endometriosis (see page 86) is also linked to infertility.

Fertility problems associated with sperm

Male fertility issues are now recognized as an equal cause in subfertility and infertility problems. Old-fashioned attitudes are being replaced by the recognition that all men can benefit from boosting their fertility. If you need a sperm count, you may be asked to undertake as many as three tests before your physician considers that any specialized investigation is needed. This time can be used to start improving your sperm quality, density, and motility through the countdown to conception program.

Sperm testing can be undertaken in privacy and with great sensitivity—in some instances using home-testing kits, There are two steps in the sperm-testing process. First, sperm are checked for their density and motility (the "sperm count"). Second, if this test sheds no light on the problem and tests on your partner reveal nothing, a postcoital test (fluid taken after intercourse) is undertaken to see if there is any underlying problem. The sperm count alone does not test for the presence of all fluids essential for fertilization. Tests will typically need to be repeated several times during your countdown to conception program to monitor your progress.

Sperm defects, or dysfunctions, are an increasing reality in modern life, yet much can be done to help men with low sperm counts or poor-quality sperm. Start by eliminating toxins, avoiding pesticides, additives, and chemicals in food, and having a healthy diet and lifestyle.

One cause of male infertility is deformed sperm. The examples in this magnified picture have misshapen heads and would be unlikely to be able to fertilize an egg.

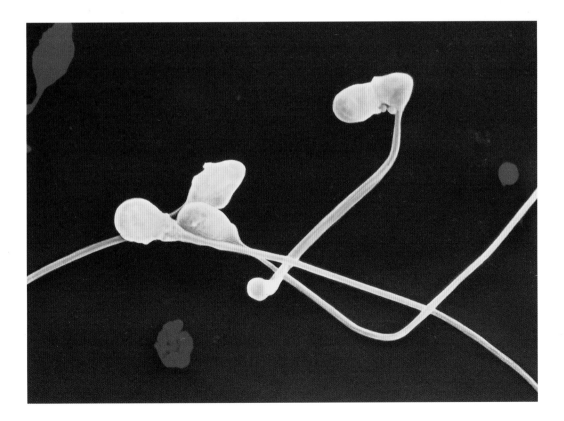

The results of sperm tests

Male fertility problems are divided into two groups:

■ **Azoospermia**: no sperm is produced by the testes.
This is very rare and is mainly associated with undescended
testicles. Some treatments for severe illnesses, such as cytotoxic
drugs or radiation therapy for cancer, can also be the cause of
this problem, and it is important to understand the significance
of embarking on such treatments, since the condition may be
irreversible later. Viral infections, such as mumps and herpes,
particularly if suffered in adolescence and beyond, can also
cause abnormalities of the testes and epididymis.

■ **Oligospermia**: sperm that is low in quantity or poor
in quality, or sometimes both.
This situation is on the increase in industrial societies.
A sperm count of 400 million is considered fertile; below
this is classified as subfertile. But conception can still be
achieved within this lower range; number alone is not the
only condition for success. In addition to improving your
nutrition and boosting your fertility, you may be advised to
take ginseng, which can increase sperm number and motility.

Some typical causes associated with oligospermia include
injury, infections, or past operations in the genital area. Problems
may also be caused by a condition known as varicocele, in which
a spermatic varicose vein becomes tight or twisted. Surgical
treatment is usually needed, and is generally successful.

Increased heat around the testes will affect sperm production,
and dramatic results can be achieved simply by removing the
causes. These include:

■ Excessively hot baths.
■ Being significantly overweight.
■ Wearing tight underwear, particularly that made from nylon
or other synthetic materials.
■ Long hours of sedentary work, such as driving.

Testing for infections

Often infections are picked up without any symptoms being
experienced, and "screening" is a way of checking for the
existence of any of these infections and viruses. They are
usually treatable and can be cleared up at an early stage
in your countdown to conception.

If an infection is found in either of you, it is likely that you will
both be treated because of the importance of eliminating such

Fertility problems
Conditions affecting male
and female fertility can have
several causes:
• Bacterial infections such
as chlamydia, which may
produce no symptoms.
• Viruses such as herpes
and AIDS.
• Anerobic bacteria such as
gardnerella.
• Deficiencies in minerals
such as zinc.

conditions. If left, they may flare up with pregnancy, affecting the mother-to-be and increasing the possibility of a premature delivery, or be passed on to your child. Examples include:

- **Chlamydia trachomatis** is the most common problem for both men and women. It often presents no symptoms, but can reduce semen quality and inflame prostate tubes in men.
- **The herpes virus** can also cause inflammation, this time of the testicles, and can lead to a low sperm count.
- **Gonorrhea**, now thankfully less common, is highly contagious and causes low sperm counts and sometimes total sterility.
- **Celiac disease** may cause gynecological and obstetric problems. It is thought to be connected to "infertility of unexplained origin," but can be detected through careful screening and treated with relaxation, nutritional and drug treatments, or a glutenfree diet.
- **Pelvic inflammatory disease** (**P.I.D.**) may cause infertility, and it is important to detect and treat it as early as possible.

There are other pelvic and genital-urinary diseases that can also have serious implications. Your clinician will advise you if he believes tests are necessary.

A healthy body will enclose viruses in a "capsid" or shell. When the immune system is low, these shells break down, releasing the virus into the body and causing illness. This picture shows a herpes simplex virus 24 hours after infection has occurred.

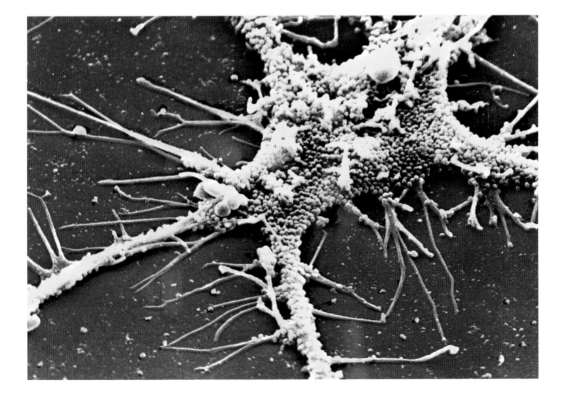

Hazards affecting fertility

Environmental hazards can seriously damage your health and fertility (see Chapter 2 pages 58–61). Here are some of the most common problems:

- Cigarette smoking reduces sperm numbers, sperm motility, and DNA quality. Chemicals that mimic estrogen, found in items such as common pesticides and household paints as well as in cigarettes, affect fertility and may be linked to cancers of the breast, ovary, and testes.
- Alcohol reduces sperm production and testosterone levels. It can also decrease your libido (the urge to have sex) and increase impotence (the inability to perform). Deficiencies in seminal fluid, caused by alcohol, can reduce the sperm motility and prevent your body from fully absorbing essential vitamins and minerals.
- Pesticides, herbicides, fungicides, and fertilizers have a direct effect on the body, particularly on the reproductive system, as well as affecting your ability to absorb important nutrients, such as vitamins and minerals. Such agrochemicals may also impair the health of your future offspring. Any action you can

Smoke warning
Research indicates that chemicals in cigarette smoke are linked to damage of the reproductive system of the baby in the womb. In male children, this may lead to low sperm counts in adult life. In girls, the chemicals can damage the egg supply and cause future miscarriages.

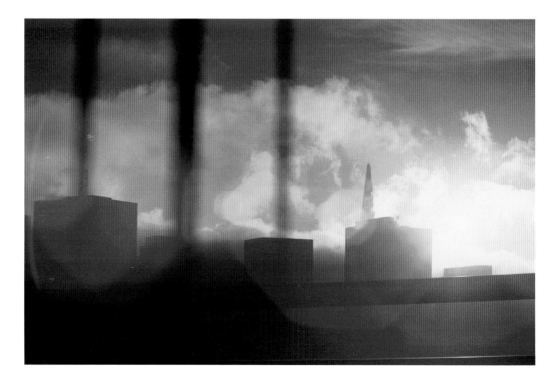

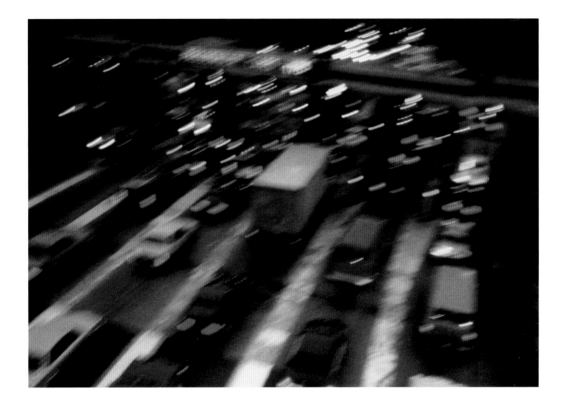

take to avoid, cut down, or cut out contact will benefit your whole family. Residues are found on fruit and vegetables as well as in drinking water, and people working in forestry and agriculture are particularly at risk.

- Chemicals that affect fertility are also found within the home. These include paint, cleaning materials, and wood-preservative treatments. New curtains and carpets also contain chemicals that can damage sperm levels.

- Food additives are found in many processed foods. They have been linked to the injury of chromosomes and genes carrying the genetic code, as well as to behavioral problems in children. Some additives also have a negative effect on the ability to absorb minerals, such as zinc, which are crucial to our wellbeing and the production of healthy offspring.

- Lead and other heavy metals used in the production of batteries and paint or absorbed through old water pipes can affect sperm count and motility, even at apparently low levels of exposure. The absorption of lead is also linked to diets deficient in minerals and vitamins, particularly calcium and vitamin C; similarly, diets high in fat and low in protein encourage lead absorption. By contrast, copper is an essential mineral, but too high a concentration in the body can lead to

Traffic-laden roads and city living may not be good for your health, but it is not always possible to move to a healthier environment. Instead, try to compensate by making your life as healthy as possible in other ways, such as having a good diet and taking plenty of exercise.

problems, particularly in areas where soft, acid water is supplied through copper pipes.

It is vital to remember that hazards do not occur in isolation. If they did, our bodies would be better equipped to eliminate them from our systems. We are now all exposed to a "cocktail" of hazards, such as food additives, pesticide residues, and chemicals in the home, at varying levels. The countdown to conception is based on a holistic and systematic approach to removing toxins by improving nutritional and absorption levels, which, in turn, will boost your fertility.

Medication and recreational drugs

There are concerns associated with any drug and its impact on fertility, whether prescribed medication, drugs bought over the counter, or "recreational" drugs. Adverse reactions can also be magnified when drugs are taken in combination.

Avoid these common medications as far as possible, but do not stop treatment regimes without consulting your doctor:

Antibiotics are commonly overprescribed, so patients become tolerant of them and the natural immune system is weakened. Since they are useless in viral illnesses, alternative remedies should be considered (see Chapter 4 for advice on alternative therapies). Antibiotics are also commonly given to animals reared for food and may pass into humans through milk and meat products. Select organic products wherever possible to avoid this risk.

Antidepressants and "beta-blockers" cause loss of libido and decreased sperm count and motility, all of which can be gradually reversed. Detoxification treatments and vitamin/ mineral supplements will help restore your health.

Diabetes medication affects fertility and is linked with birth defects. You may benefit from vitamin and mineral supplements to help you to reduce your insulin dependency.

Epilepsy medication: treatment regimes should be addressed. Mineral deficiencies and chemical additives linked to epilepsy can be helped by dietary guidance.

Painkillers, particularly opiates, deplete hormones that trigger sperm development.

Heroin and LSD are neurotoxins that alter behavior by affecting brain function. Heroin use decreases testosterone and leads to reduced fertility in men. In women, it increases the chances of complications in pregnancy.

Antihistamines are commonly prescribed or available over the counter. While they help to reduce hay fever symptoms, they can also interfere with fluid levels in the body. Seek help to reduce the underlying causes of hay fever allergies by using homeopathic remedies or nutritional therapy, and by making lifestyle changes.

Cannabis use is believed to lower testosterone levels and sperm counts and can reduce libido and increase impotency in men. It also upsets the female menstrual cycle and can prolong or even stop labor.

Avoiding fertility hazards

Avoid	Why?	Benefits
Alcohol	Alcohol reduces: • The ability to perform and enjoy sex. • Sperm strength and movement.	Avoiding alcohol: • Improves digestion. • Improves absorption of foods, vitamins, and minerals.
Chemicals in food and water and around the home	• Chemicals deplete trace minerals in food, notably zinc, manganese, iron, magnesium, and potassium. • Chemicals can cause impotency and birth defects. • Chemicals can cause cancer.	• Improves levels of trace minerals in the body, such as zinc for sperm development and manganese for muscle tone.
Food additives	• They cause food intolerance or "allergies." • They cause birth defects and child behavioral problems; they injure chromosomes and genes before conception.	• Fewer migraines, hay fever, skin, and digestive problems. • Improves your future child's chances of good health.

Chapter four

Complementary care

Ancient wisdom sees conception as a joyous and important occasion: a precious opportunity to create a new and unique life. Traditional health-care systems from around the world stress the importance of this moment in determining the character and wellbeing of the future child.

Scientific research has also shown that the parents' health makes a difference to the genetic qualities that are passed on to their child. It is vital, therefore, for you to boost your wellbeing in preparation for conception and to be happy and relaxed at this special time.

Complementary health care can make a life-enhancing contribution to preconceptional care. This chapter describes the range of holistic complementary treatments now available—and increasingly integrated into orthodox health care. The approach of these systems may differ, but all aim to strengthen the body, cleanse the system, and stimulate self-healing mechanisms. The human body is seen as sensitive, intelligent matter that can be encouraged to regain balance and heal itself.

Traditional Chinese medicine, for example, which describes the life force as "chi," or "qi," energy, talks about a creative substance called "jing," which is the constitutional health passed on to us from our parents at conception. Ayurvedic medicine recommends a purification program for future parents, based on their constitutions; it also relates these constitutions, known as *doshas*, to certain seasons when it is better to attempt, or refrain from attempting, conception.

Complementary health care can enhance fertility and support the clinical care couples receive. It is important, though, that practitioners have experience in fertility issues and that they are qualified in their therapies and accredited to a professional body. These checks will reassure both you and your physician.

Typically, a practitioner will offer advice on nutrition, lifestyle, and relaxation, as well as proposing a treatment or remedy. Most importantly, holistic methods promote responsible self-care, encouraging a healthy body, mind, and spirit. These complementary therapies can offer invaluable care and practical support to you both during your countdown to conception.

A gentle massage is a perfect way of relaxing and relieving stress during your countdown to conception. Book regular appointments for yourself and your partner, and learn some of the simpler techniques for use at home.

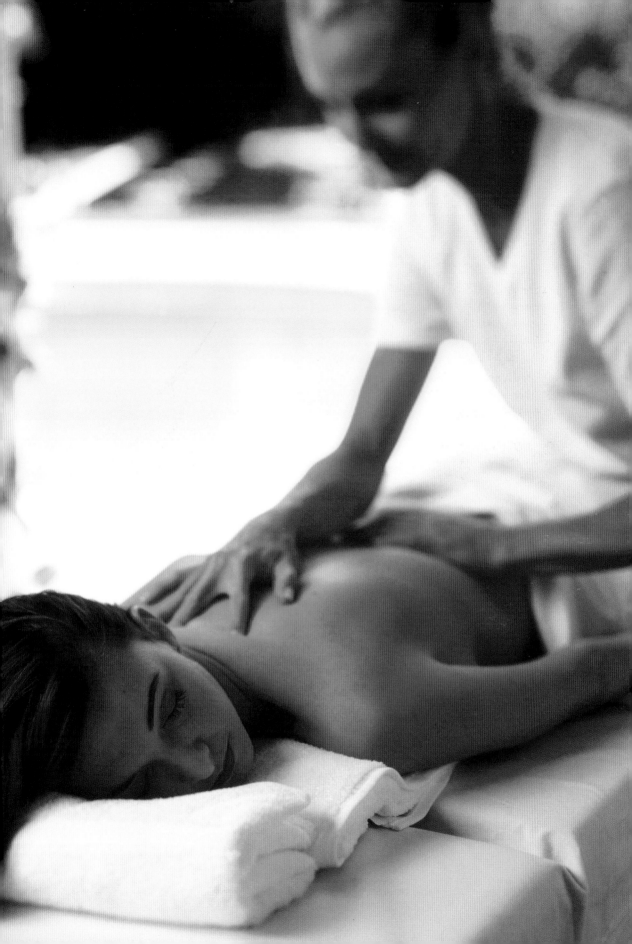

In this chapter you will find a variety of complementary approaches from different cultures. Knowledge of the power of herbs, oils, and essences dates back thousands of years in China and India, for example, and evidence of similar knowledge has been found in ancient Egyptian texts. Today, people are becoming more and more interested in these traditional therapies, as well as in more recent ones such as homeopathy.

Movement therapies such as yoga, t'ai chi, and chi kung are examples of ancient eastern exercises now widely practiced in the West. More recently developed treatments to improve our posture and reduce wear and tear on our spine, such as the Alexander technique, osteopathy, and chiropractic, are increasingly recognized by the medical profession as valuable.

If you have a specific diagnosed condition, complementary approaches to health care may help to reduce your medication, eradicate unwanted side-effects, and improve your symptoms. Use holistic techniques to complement your medical advice, but make sure your doctor is aware of your integrated approach. This way, you will avoid the risks associated with sudden breaks in medication, or inappropriate treatments.

Success with homeopathy

This is a true story, told to me by a couple with a history of fertility problems.

Julie had suffered early and particularly heavy periods, as well as problems with endometriosis and a double uterus. She and her husband Russell had been trying for a family for more than ten years when Julie was referred to a fertility clinic. She conceived at the first attempt, but lost the child at nine weeks. Julie and Russell decided to give up IVF after the third attempt. The stress had been so great that they put aside all thoughts of having children.

Julie first consulted a homeopath for help with her periods, which were increasingly heavy, with midterm bleeding. After two treatments, Julie told Andrew, her homeopath, that she and Russell were reconsidering a "last chance" attempt at IVF, using her stored eggs. Andrew recommended that she first try a homeopathic remedy, based on a natural hormone secreted in the ovary. The remedy is used in a wide range of hormonal problems, including endometriosis and polycystic ovary syndrome, as well as to increase fertility. "I told Julie that she would need treatment over about six months to be successful," said Andrew. "But I was wrong! I received a letter from her in June saying she had conceived naturally after her last treatment in April and was now ten weeks pregnant."

This story has a classic happy ending. Julie and Russell's son Samuel was born at 35 weeks, weighing 5½ pounds. Although he was a little on the small side, Samuel is healthy and seems determined to catch up soon!

Take care with complementary therapies

In the hands of a qualified and experienced practitioner, complementary therapies and medicines are generally enjoyable and extremely safe. Health is about a balanced lifestyle, and if you have a problem, your practitioner will be looking for areas of imbalance in your life: these may be in your diet, your lifestyle, or your psychological wellbeing.

Holistic health care works on the principle of improving your total wellbeing, instead of just addressing individual symptoms, and is particularly beneficial for couples preparing for pregnancy. Always tell your practitioners that you are planning to conceive and warn them if you believe you may already be pregnant, since there are particular oils, herbs, yoga positions, and meridian points that should be avoided at this time. Do tell your practitioners if you have a history of miscarriage or other preexisting health conditions.

If you are seeking a practitioner for the first time, there are some important questions to ask about their training, accreditation, and experience. The reference section at the back of this book lists sources of help in finding a practitioner. If you have not experienced a particular therapy before, ask your practitioner to describe the way he or she works, how long each treatment will take, and what sort of effects you might expect. Give yourself time after a treatment to "come to." Don't rush home and do anything strenuous. Drinking alcohol or even making love may counteract all the benefits. Relax for the rest of the day, and let the treatment keep on working through your system.

Sometimes symptoms may appear to get worse before they get better, particularly if an illness has been progressing for some time. This may show as tiredness, a rash, a cough, or other symptoms. Using nutritional therapy or reflexology to cleanse your system of toxins, for example, may stimulate symptoms as your body "flushes out" toxic material. Complementary therapies are not instant cures, and preexisting conditions may continue for a while before the treatment encourages your body's self-healing mechanisms to take over. For example, if you start a course of vitamins or minerals, they will take up to 30 days to become absorbed at cellular level.

Keep your physician informed
You are advised to keep your physician informed of your decision to use a complementary practitioner, particularly if you have a preexisting condition such as high blood pressure, diabetes, or epilepsy. Tell your physician if you plan to adopt a special diet that means restricting certain foods, and take great care not to cut out medication suddenly or without advice.

Your clinician needs to take into account possible interactions between treatments, and communication between professionals is very important. For example, if you are following a course of nutritional supplements you might consider asking your therapist to write a letter to your clinician, explaining his or her qualifications and experience, as well as the rationale behind the treatment. Many practitioners are trained in the special needs of couples who wish to conceive, and their recommendations should take precedence over those of therapists who are not qualified in nutritional medicine.

Shared information may cut down on the number of tests you need and may speed up your countdown. With your permission, good communication between your physician and complementary practitioner is always helpful.

Distilling the essence

The use of diluted or concentrated natural substances, such as the roots, leaves, or flowers of plants, has been proven to encourage the body's own natural defenses against illness. Treatments range from the physical application of oils through aromatherapy massage to the subtle use of flower essences.

Aromatherapy

Essential oils have been used since Egyptian times to heal sickness. They are concentrated by a distillation process and absorbed through the skin or by inhalation. Oils are deeply sensual and have a great affinity with fertility. They can help stimulate or relax us and can be used, in an oil base, on the skin or dropped into a warm bath.

An aromatherapist uses massage with essential oils to help relieve tension, improve circulation, and stimulate hormonal balance. A trained practitioner can help to select oils that will address mental, physical, and spiritual ailments, restoring hormonal and psychological balance. If there is any possibility that you might already be pregnant when you go for an aromatherapy treatment, be sure to tell your therapist. There are certain volatile oils that must be avoided in pregnancy.

Flower essences

Flower essence remedies are an ancient method of healing, rediscovered in England by Dr. Edward Bach more than 60 years ago. The use of his 38 Bach Flower Remedies is based on the principle that flower essences help to restore harmony in cases of negative states of mind that can lead to illness. Following his work, other practitioners around the world have harnessed the energies of other plants and flowers to stimulate healing in response to our complex needs. An Australian naturopath, for example, developed the Australian Bush Flower Essences to make use of the healing powers of flowers in his native land. These include essences such as "She Oak," which soothes the distress associated with infertility, and "Turkey Bush," which releases creativity—and thus potency—in men.

Flower essences are good for underlying emotional and psychological states, including worry, anxiety, and fear; they do not directly treat physical symptoms. Instead, they stimulate aspects of

Plants and flowers have long been linked with healing, and their properties have been recognized for thousands of years. Today, they are used to make many homeopathic remedies, as well as essential oils and flower remedies. Homeopathic and flower essence remedies are safe to give to adults, children, pets, and even plants.

the self-healing process. Many practitioners of other therapies use and recommend flower remedies in conjunction with their other treatments.

Homeopathy

Based on the principle of "like cures like," homeopathy treats patients by giving minute quantities of a substance that would cause similar symptoms in a healthy person. This stimulates the body to heal itself. Substances are "potentized" to energize the healing process. Be prepared for a homeopath to ask very detailed, searching questions—anything from the state of your health to psychological information. This will enable the practitioner to build up an individual assessment and decide on the right remedies.

Homeopathy is good for most conditions, except mechanical back problems and severe physical injury. If you suffer from a chronic condition or need help with infertility, make sure that your homeopath is qualified and experienced in these areas.

Therapies to move you

For all movement therapies, explain your plans for conception and let your teacher know if you have any particular medical conditions that may prevent you performing certain sequences or exercises. Once you have mastered a series of t'ai chi postures, yoga asanas, or Alexander technique movements, you can practice them at your leisure in your own home. At the same time, keep going to classes or follow up with occasional refresher classes. This will help you make sure you are performing the exercises correctly and that the benefits are sustained.

T'ai Chi

In this ancient exercise system, a series of fluid, graceful movements is performed to balance the flow of "chi"—or life force. The movements are so gentle, almost like a slow dance, that they can be practiced well into old age. They can be performed in short, or longer sequences. Your t'ai chi teacher can also show you specific exercises for particular conditions.

T'ai chi is good for enhancing vitality, improving balance, and inducing relaxation. If you are having problems giving up smoking, for example, t'ai chi will concentrate and calm your mind. It will enhance your overall wellbeing, rather than treat particular ailments.

Yoga

Yoga is a complete system of mind, body, and spiritual exercises, leading to the integration and balance of all parts of the body. The yoga postures, or asanas, stretch and relax the body, using breathing techniques in harmony with gentle movements. The breath or "prana" contains our vital life force, and controlled yogic breathing can help promote a relaxed state, reducing blood pressure and improving the circulation.

Yoga is a good exercise to learn when you are planning for a healthy conception—it can reduce menstrual problems, help you to prepare for pregnancy, and will become an invaluable part of your postnatal exercise regime. It stimulates and regulates hormone production and improves reproductive disorders. Special postures

Gentle movement therapies such as yoga will stimulate your circulation and improve your energy levels, confidence, and sexual function. Some asanas should be avoided during menstruation and pregnancy, so it is important to find an experienced yoga teacher who can help you develop a suitable routine.

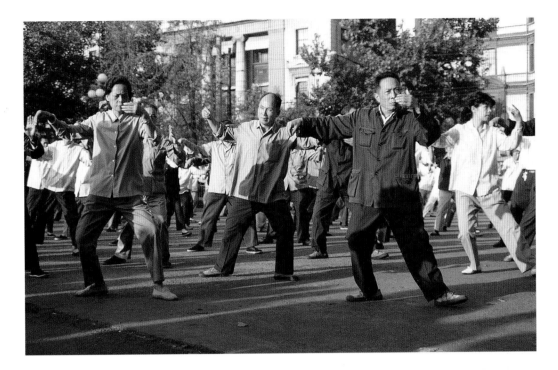

can be learned which focus on particular parts of the body that may need help. Once you conceive, you may be able to find a class that caters specially for pregnant women.

T'ai chi even exercises muscles you didn't know you had! The movements help to improve stamina, balance, and sleep problems.

Chi Kung

Often described as "exercising while standing still," chi kung is a series of exercises, combined with breathing, postures, and movements, which can treat many conditions. Chi kung is a balance of movement and rest, and is remarkably gentle, yet beneficial to the body.

In addition to benefiting your overall wellbeing, a chi kung master can guide you toward exercises or postures to help with particular problems, including acute stress, asthma, and lack of sleep, as well as chronic ailments such as digestive disorders and sexual dysfunction.

Alexander Technique

This is a process of "unlearning" bad postural habits and developing new postures that put minimum strain on the body. The Alexander Technique is good for any back or musculoskeletal problems, as well as for poor breathing or digestive problems developed as a result of poor posture. Patients are encouraged to reeducate themselves as to their posture and movements under the guidance of an expert.

Channelling your "chi" energy

Eastern medicines are based on the idea that there is a flow of energy within everyone. An invisible life force, known as "chi," passes along channels or "meridians" in the body. When these channels become blocked—or overstimulated—imbalance and poor health result. Typically integrated within a wider treatment regime of exercise, relaxation, and herbal medicine, therapies such as acupuncture and shiatsu address the whole person's needs, restoring balance and vitality.

When you go for a consultation with an acupuncturist or other complementary practitioner. you may be surprised at the amount of time the therapist spends asking questions about your lifestyle before discussing your particular condition. Holistic health care approaches generally examine psychological as well as physical symptoms. Your therapist will look at underlying causes of poor health and will, typically, ask you about your diet and your intake of alcohol and other beverages.

Acupuncture

Acupuncture has been practiced in China for more than three thousand years, as part of Traditional Chinese Medicine (TCM). It involves the stimulation of certain points on the meridians of the body, usually with fine needles. Your acupuncturist may also use "moxa," a mixture of pungent herbs burned over particular acupuncture points, to increase the benefit of your treatment.

Based on the principle of an interaction between opposite energies of "yin" and "yang," acupuncture stimulates, unblocks, or calms the energy, in response to your individual needs. Headaches and migraines can be improved, for example, by unblocking chi and stimulating the natural painkillers, or endorphins in the body.

In the West, acupuncture is now particularly recognized for its important role in the relief of discomfort for conditions such as painful periods. It is also noted for the treatment of nausea in early pregnancy. Acupuncture can also target particular meridians that will stimulate hormone production, so helping with male and female fertility problems.

Shiatsu or Acupressure

Based on a Japanese approach to meridian points, shiatsu uses physical pressure, rather than needles, to treat different energy points. Practitioners may use their fingers or thumbs, even sometimes elbows, feet or knees, to apply pressure. This may

Pelvic floor exercise
Eastern medicine describes sexual dysfunction as an excess of yin over yang energy. Try this exercise every day to recharge your sexual energy.
1 Lie on your back, with your knees bent, feet on the ground and buttocks slightly raised.
2 Alternately contract and release the muscles in the perineum (in women between the anus and vagina and in men between the scrotum and anus) as if you were trying to hold back your urine.
3 Breathe deeply, inhaling while you contract and hold the muscles taut for a count of three; exhale as you gently release.
4 Repeat daily up to 60 times or for five minutes.

sound painful but feels like a very deep massage. Practitioners will pay particular attention to your responses to treatment and may ask questions about your sleeping patterns as well as matters such as diet and exercise.

Shiatsu is a whole-body balance, massaging, energizing, or relaxing you to address your particular physical needs. If you have an underlying health problem, such as chronic fatigue or a low immune system, regular shiatsu treatments can bring your body back into balance. Shiatsu is also particularly useful for releasing tension and for restoring the body's natural hormonal system after coming off the pill. Your practitioner may also show you self-help techniques that you can use at home to ease your symptoms in between treatments.

This patient is undergoing acupuncture treatment for hay fever, with needles inserted into certain points just under the skin. Such therapies can be extremely successful and can help you avoid taking medication during your countdown to conception.

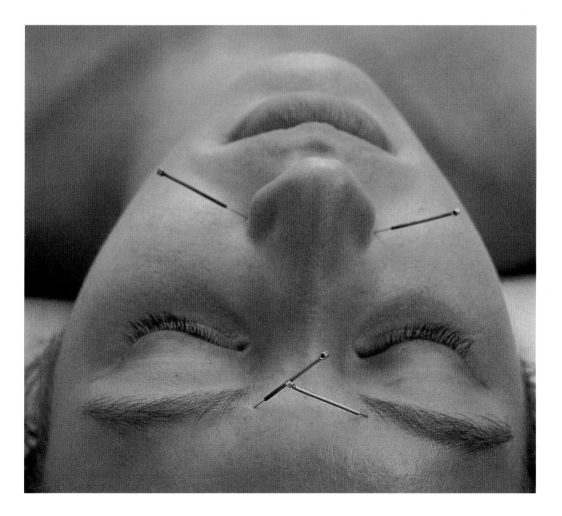

Nutritional and herbal therapies

Nutritional and herbal therapists can help your body's own healing systems by improving your nutrition and recommending specific herbal remedies. These systems are based on the key principle that the body, given enough support, can heal itself. To get the most benefit from treatment, you may need to make some changes to your lifestyle over a period of time.

Always consult a qualified practitioner. Although derived from natural ingredients, many herbs have powerful properties and should be prescribed only by professionals. While some common herbs are ideal for self-help use, others should be treated with caution, particularly when planning pregnancy.

Your practitioner may advise a complete nutritional regime, which should be continued at home long after treatment for a specific problem ceases. These therapies treat the whole person, and will benefit most conditions, including digestive, sexual, and hormonal problems.

Naturopathy

A naturopathic treatment typically begins by detoxifying your system, often using raw and whole foods and water; fasting may also be recommended. You will be encouraged to take your cooked foods simply—without highly salted or spiced sauces. A regime of nutritional therapy is then proposed, often using supplements to boost your immune system and prevent illness.

The naturopath will suggest foods that provide the nutritional, vitamin, and mineral elements that you lack. For example, women suffering from premenstrual dizziness may be advised to eat large amounts of parsley and watercress to increase iron levels in an easily digestible form. Oats are an accessible source of nutrition and have a stimulating effect on men suffering from impotence.

Chinese herbal medicine and food cures

Chinese medicine arises out of several different approaches
to health care, dating back thousands of years. The treatments
available in the West are just a fraction of the vast expertise that
exists. In Chinese medicine, food has five flavors; five energies
are generated by foods; and there are four "movements." These
principles are then considered in conjunction with your body
type—how yin or yang you are, and how well your chi is flowing.

Chinese herbs typically use five active ingredients in a
complex mix, specially balanced for your condition. The mixing
of different herbs avoids unwanted side-effects and accords
with the principles of the five elements. Food cures will often
combine common foods in "recipes" to address specific ailments.

Western herbalism

Western herbal medicine also has a long history and is in
sympathy with eastern concepts of strengthening the body's vital
force. As in Chinese herbalism, the complex principle of "active
constituents" applies, with different constituents, typically
within one plant, working together in harmony. Different parts
of the plant may be used—including seeds, bark, flowers, and
berries—for different conditions or treatment methods.

Ayurveda

Like traditional Chinese medicine, ayurveda is part of an
ancient system of holistic healing. It dates back to ancient
Hindu teachings, which link health with physical,
mental, and spiritual wellbeing.

Diagnosis is based on an analysis of your attributes, based
on the three vital energies or *doshas*. Imbalances of *doshas* disrupt
the life force and cause the symptom associated with illness.

Ayurvedic teaching also emphasizes the importance of
living in harmony with the seasons and recommends that
conception takes place at the time of year most
suitable to your *doshas*, insuring your
wellbeing and that of your future child.

Treatment may include herbs, oils,
and other supplements, as well as cleansing
and detoxifying therapy; relaxation
techniques are also important.

*By improving your overall wellbeing,
nutritional and herbal therapies can
help many conditions that may affect
your fertility, including migraines, and
digestive and circulatory problems.
They treat the reproductive system very
effectively, easing period problems and
improving sex drive and sperm count.*

Some tried and tested remedies

Name and description	Benefit
Aloe vera gel Antifungal treatment	Restores the digestive system, relieves menstrual cramps. Caution: do not take if you are pregnant or breastfeeding.
Acidophilus Increases "friendly" gut bacteria	Combats yeast infections such as candida; improves the ability to absorb nutrients; particularly useful for diabetics.
Echinacea Boosts the immune system	Aids recovery from repeated colds or flu; improves overall wellbeing.
Evening primrose Contains essential fatty acids (EFAs)	Good for menstrual problems; improves skin conditions; helps ease discomfort of tender breasts prior to a period.
Feverfew Reduces levels of serotonin, a hormone that triggers migraines	Prevents migraine; brings on delayed periods; relieves period pains and PMT.
Garlic Antibacterial and antiviral properties	Strongly antibiotic; lowers blood pressure and reduces cholesterol and fat levels, improves circulation.
Ginger Relaxant for intestines	Promotes menstruation, alleviates nausea, relaxes muscle spasm. Invigorates the reproductive system.
Ginseng Contains natural testosterone	Stimulates sexual dysfunction in both men and women. Helps to reverse impotence.
Ginkgo biloba Improves circulatory system	Reduces mood swings, improves mental clarity, helps to reverse impotence.
Live yogurt Antiviral and antifungal treatment	Restores digestive bacteria following use of antibiotics. Treatment for candida infection and herpes virus.
St. John's Wort Muscle relaxant	Relieves menstrual problems: painful, heavy, and irregular periods and PMT. Excellent for anxiety and depression.
Saw palmetto Nourishes sex organs	Helps low libido and impotence in men and good for inflamed and enlarged prostate. Relieves painful periods.
Tea tree Antibacterial and antifungal	Relieves the symptoms of many infections such as cold sores and genital herpes.

Massage and manipulation therapies

Massage is one of the easiest techniques to learn and use at home. Even gently rubbing your partner's hands or feet can be deeply soothing. Some techniques require great skill, helping to heal painful and chronic conditions. Manipulative therapies, for example, should never be attempted at home, and you should be treated only by a professional practitioner.

However, you may be given some exercises to continue, or be recommended herbs or oils suitable for home use. Remember to tell your practitioner that you are planning to conceive. Some treatments should not be attempted if you might be pregnant, and there are certain volatile oils that should be avoided.

Massage

Massage can be deeply relaxing, helping to improve the circulation and alleviate muscle pain. There are many different techniques, and some therapists concentrate on a single part of the body—just massaging your hands with the right oils can be beneficial, and Indian head massage is relaxing and uplifting.

Don't be fooled by the gentle touch of massage; it can have a very powerful effect, lasting for days after your treatment, and can help your body eliminate toxins. By relaxing your neck and lower spine, massage can help your posture and self-confidence over the longer term. If your stress comes from overexertion and physical causes, massage relaxes you. By learning a few simple massage techniques, you can also improve your relationship— giving a massage is a perfect way to express affection.

Reflexology

Each organ and area of your body is represented on the feet, and reflexology uses point pressure to prevent and cure disorders in other parts of the body. An ancient therapy, it has been developed as a diagnostic tool and treatment for physical and emotional problems, and is particularly successful in treating fertility and menstrual problems. Reflexology may also be used to detoxify your system generally by improving your circulation.

Chiropractic and Osteopathy

The manipulative therapies, such as osteopathy and chiropractic, focus on the musculoskeletal system, and the interaction of bones, joints, and muscles. They are very effective for such conditions as back pain, trapped nerves, or migraine, all of which may be underlying factors preventing conception.

Lavender
Some very common garden plants have valuable properties. Lavender is a natural, all-round antiseptic. It also relaxes brain waves; can help to relieve stress, anxiety, and panic attacks; and stimulates tissue repair. You can even make a non-toxic household cleaner from lavender.

Healing from within

Don't forget to nourish your inner self. You will benefit from the appreciation of the real value of life and the importance of living each day in touch with your feelings and needs—regardless of what the day brings.

Healing

Most complementary practitioners will take a holistic approach to their patients' needs, including healing body, mind, and spirit. Some practitioners will consider the spiritual level first, addressing the need to be at peace as a priority. Feeling positive —even in the presence of illness—will help to diminish symptoms, since so many flare up when you are under stress.

The concept of a healing life force is important to understanding the healing process, and many practitioners will use this energy, without calling themselves "healers." Being open to healing does not involve religious or spiritual belief, although some practitioners feel that their skill is a God-given power.

Meditation

Simple meditation can take many forms and be practiced wherever you can find a quiet corner and have time to give to yourself. Instead of expending your energy by looking outward at external experiences, it helps you turn within and find inner calm. Regular practice will help you stay more relaxed and less vulnerable to stress and tension.

You can focus on an object, such as a candle, listen to gentle background music, chant a mantra, or repeat a phrase silently to yourself. Concentrating on your breathing is another simple technique. How profound or deep your experience is will depend partly on the amount of time and concentration you are able to give, and how regularly you can practice.

The purpose is to quieten your mind and improve your focus and concentration. The effect is like a "wakeful sleep," which generates relaxing "alpha" rhythms in your brainwave pattern. Initially, you may feel like lying down and falling asleep; if this is what your body needs, then listen and do it.

Sometimes meditation brings anxiety, anger, and other emotions to the surface, particularly if they have been repressed for years. Physical activity, such as a brisk walk, will dissipate these tensions and help channel your newfound energy. Do speak to a professional counselor or meditation teacher, however, if these feelings continue and are a cause of concern.

An energy booster
For a quick visualization, when you're feeling out of balance or needing a boost of energy, picture the infinity sign—a figure eight on its side. Follow its lines from left to right and back again and then right to left. Do this with your eyes open and then with them closed. This will quickly refresh you and rebalance your left and right brain hemispheres.
If an image surfaces that disturbs or upsets you, remember it is just your imagination trying to express an idea. Talk it over with your partner and, if you would like professional guidance, speak to your doctor or a trained counselor.

Creative visualization

Visualization is an excellent way of relaxing and accessing your subconscious. You can practice it alone or with your partner, taking turns to read out the instructions, pausing whenever necessary. Some people are quicker at visualizing than others, but take your own time and don't be rushed. Before you start, plan your goal. If you want to boost your fertility, there may be a key word or image you can use to sum up your aim. When you find it, you're ready to start.

1 Find a quiet place to sit and relax. Breathe slowly, keeping both feet on the floor. When you are ready, close your eyes and imagine energy coming up through your legs from the ground, revitalizing you to the tips of your fingers and the top of your head. This is a basic energizing exercise, and you can stop here if you want.

2 Now for a relaxing visualization. Imagine your ideal environment—perhaps sitting beside the sea, or a gently moving river. Picture the scene, building up the detail piece by piece: the birds moving between branches, flowers blossoming near the ground. Some people can even hear the sounds, picture the colors, and imagine the smells. This is your place of peace and tranquility, where you can go for mental respite and return refreshed to your everyday world.

3 If you are ready to move on, just keep your eyes closed and focus on your particular issue. Can you give it a picture?

- To help build up sperm, picture them as active, growing things, ready to leap into life.
- For healthy eggs, you may see a gentler image, such as a bud bursting into bloom.
- To help combat an infection, visualize burning it on a fire, or find some other mental image that kills the illness.
- To reach out for support and friendship, imagine your soul mates as trees in a wood, protecting each other, or as lighthouses throwing out rays to ships in distress.
- If you want to cut the ties from your past, you might imagine a ribbon and a pair of scissors—the official opening of your new life!

4 When you have found the right image for your situation, sit and watch it taking place—under your control. Build up the image until you are enacting the situation in your imagination.

5 When you are ready to finish, come to by feeling the weight of your limbs. In your own time, open your eyes and get used to your surroundings again. Stretch and stand up.

Use complementary therapies to help...

Give up addictions

Complementary approaches are good for addictive habits, such as drinking alcohol, taking drugs, or even eating chocolate. Remember that an addiction is a psychological issue, as well as a problem affecting your physical health. It may also indicate a nutritional imbalance.

Acupuncture can ease withdrawal symptoms; yoga relaxes and helps boost self-confidence; hypnotherapy is a tried and tested positive approach to giving up smoking. Visualizations and relaxation tapes may help calm your mind and nerves.

Stabilize diabetes

When planning to conceive, the aim is to balance blood sugar levels naturally and to improve overall wellbeing, while cutting down on medication that may affect the health of your future child. Seek your doctor's advice on holistic approaches and do not stop taking medication, although you may be able to reduce it as your system rebalances itself.

Your nutritionist or naturopath may recommend a diet high in unrefined carbohydrates to improve your pancreatic function, balance your blood sugar level, and cleanse your digestive system. Brown rice, for example, stabilizes insulin and blood sugar levels.

Herbal remedies to reduce blood sugar levels may help, as will specific vitamin and mineral supplements such as vitamin C and chromium. Reflexology techniques can help improve circulation, as well as work on the liver, pancreas, and pituitary glands. Relaxation, yoga, and meditation may all help increase blood flow and reduce the need for insulin.

Reduce anxiety and stress

Meditation, relaxation, stress management, and breathing techniques reduce anxiety, relax muscles, and improve an impaired immune system. Find a technique that suits you, like daily relaxation exercises or coping techniques for stressful situations and anxiety or asthma attacks. Hypertension, high blood pressure, and migraines can all be reduced.

For fatigue caused by long-term stress or depression, massage and aromatherapy treat deep muscle tension and lift your spirits. Bergamot, lavender, rose, and ylang-ylang are all beneficial for preconceptional care. Homeopathy can identify and treat underlying anxiety. Yoga postures are used to relax the body and expand the lungs.

Relieve discomfort from menstruation

Restore normal hormone balance with a high-fiber diet, including essential fatty acids. Herbs such as evening primrose and camomile tea can help to regulate hormones and improve liver function. Irregular periods can be treated with herbs, aromatherapy, and essential oils, which will help induce menstruation. If premenstrual syndrome is a recurring problem and includes the craving for foods such as chocolate, nutritional therapy will help, and cramps and tenderness can be treated with herbal remedies. Relieve stress with gentle exercise, relaxation, and visualization techniques.

Eradicate candidiasis

The excessive growth of the yeastlike fungus *Candida albicans* is now a common problem, largely due to overuse of antibiotics and the pill. Stress and nutritional problems may exacerbate the disorder, causing problems such as chronic fatigue, irritability, and digestive problems. It is important to clear up candida before you become pregnant, since it may worsen during pregnancy.

Where stress is a trigger, symptoms can be helped by relaxation and breathing techniques, combined with massage or acupuncture treatments to improve the digestion and regulate bowel function.

A naturopath may recommend cutting out all yeast-based products from the diet, including beer and refined foods, because the fungus feeds on the starch and sugar. Yogurts containing live organisms, such as acidophilus, are often recommended to restore the natural digestive bacteria that keep candida in check. Herbal remedies—douches, tinctures, and essential oils—may all be prescribed.

Deal with hay fever

Cutting down on antihistamine treatments may help boost your fertility. Avoid additives, wheat, and dairy products, including cow's milk, cheese, milk chocolate, and other mucus-inducing foods. Switching to organic milk may help if your sensitivity is to the unwanted additives in non-organic milk.

Homeopathic remedies and acupuncture can help to ease hay fever, or try aromatherapy treatments with lavender, lemon balm, and eucalyptus oil. For blocked sinuses, use eucalyptus and tea tree. Naturopathy can help identify the allergens, eliminate them, and boost your immune system.

Minimize the symptoms of multiple sclerosis

Good nutritional levels will help you to reduce the symptoms and flare-ups of MS. You should also take advice about the possibility of any food allergies or intolerances—removing these may improve your symptoms. This will also help to boost your immune system, making you less vulnerable to infection and improving your libido and fertility.

Lack of sensation, fatigue, or low self-confidence may diminish your sex drive. Try some of the visualization and relaxation tips on pages 110–111 and learn massage techniques that stimulate your energy.

As long as you pace your activities carefully, exercise is often recommended and should be combined with plenty of rest.

Minimize digestive problems

Your digestion is the first line of defense against illness and is the first point of absorption of nutrients. Untreated celiac disease, for example, may be responsible for "unexplained infertility." An allergy to wheat or gluten (also found in barley, rye, and oats) can cause an intolerance in the small intestine that renders it unable to absorb nutrients from food. Typical symptoms include tiredness, loss of weight, and a feeling of weakness.

Irritable bowel syndrome, or IBS, may also be a reaction to certain foods or additives or due to a lack of fiber in the diet. Symptoms often include alternating diarrhea and constipation. If you have any undiagnosed or unexplained symptoms, seek help from a qualified nutritionist.

Check the growth of fibroids

Fibroids are non-malignant growths on the lining of the womb that may prevent conception. Caused by an imbalance of estrogen, which is stored in fat, fibroids may cause heavy prolonged periods, prevent conception, and obstruct childbirth. Use massage and yoga to improve circulation in the pelvic area. Eliminate excess estrogen by changing to a low-fat, high-fiber diet, rich in whole grains and fresh fruit.

Contain herpes viruses

Viruses are agents that can only grow or reproduce within living cells. Once we are infected by certain viruses, they remain in our bodies for life. Normally they exist within the body covered by a protein shell, or capsid, which contains the virus and prevents it from proliferating.

The herpes virus is a common infection which causes painful blisters either on the face (type 1) or the genitals (type 2). When the immune system is lowered, the virus is activated and will spread.

Outbreaks are also connected with high stress levels and can erupt during or just before menstruation.

It is important to boost your overall immune levels to avoid problems during pregnancy. Nutritional improvements, including vitamin and mineral therapy, will help reduce outbreaks. If they do occur, essential oils such as tea tree can help, as can bathing in dilutions of herbs such as lemon balm.

Prevent sexual dysfunction and loss of libido

A lack of interest in sex can sometimes be the result of an infection or medication for a preexisting problem, and medical help should be sought immediately to rule this out. If back pain is the cause of the problem, this should be checked with a chiropractor or osteopath.

Hormonal imbalances—notably a deficiency of testosterone—can be the underlying cause of loss of libido in both men and women. Avoid meat that is not from organic sources, since estrogen is used to increase animal growth artificially and is passed through the food chain. A general lack of zinc or other vitamins and minerals may be part of the problem. Zinc helps to restore libido and improve a man's erection.

New medications, such as Viagra, may be a temporary solution if medically prescribed. A holistic approach will help restore sexual function naturally over the longer term so you are not reliant on drugs. This may include the use of some of the remedies suggested on page 108.

If sex is painful, it may be a sign that there is an underlying infection or a response to stress, which is another common cause of sexual problems. Premature ejaculation creates pressure on both partners; if stress is the cause, relaxation techniques, yoga, aromatherapy, and massage may all be of benefit. If your nutrition levels are low, this may also be causing sexual dysfunction.

Homeopathy has an excellent record in treating male sexual problems such as impotence, and ginseng and other supplements can help boost testosterone levels. Other helpful treatments include acupuncture and shiatsu, or acupressure to stimulate meridian energy.

Massage will increase erogenous arousal and essential oils, such as ylang-ylang, will improve the libido and can be used together with jasmine, lavender, or rose oils to relax the body and stimulate sensuality.

Alleviate endometriosis

Endometriosis (see page 86) is a painful condition caused by menstrual tissue migrating outside the womb and clinging to other points in the body. The tissue continues to grow and bleed, as if it were still in the womb.

Under careful supervision, nutritional and herbal medicine can help greatly relieve symptoms and improve the chances of conception. Supplements such as evening primrose oil can be of particular benefit if estrogen levels are high. Treatment for candidiasis may also be necessary.

Reduce headaches and migraines

While the causes of these two conditions are the same—stress coupled with neck and shoulder tension—the effects are markedly different. The frightening symptoms of migraines can create a cycle of anxiety and pain.

Migraine triggers can include stimulants such as coffee, tea, and colas containing caffeine; missed meals, causing blood sugar swings; loss of sleep or too little exercise. If you use a computer for your job, check your posture and avoid eyestrain; drink plenty of water—up to four pints per day—to avoid dehydration.

Some attacks are linked to food triggers, such as cheese or chocolate. Avoiding these foods will help, as will vitamin/mineral supplements. A nutritionist will help you identify your particular food triggers.

Self-help includes improving your lifestyle and taking more exercise, particularly out in the fresh air. This will, in turn, benefit your sleep patterns and enable you to feel less affected by stress.

Cope with thyroid problems

If you have hypothyroidism, the glands that produce hormones are underactive, and you may be suffering from an excess of estrogen, which can be serious. You may feel tired and depressed, have weight problems, or suffer premenstrual syndrome. Do ask your physician for a thyroid test. If untreated, this condition can lead to breast and endometrial cancer in later life.

The typical treatment from complementary practitioners will be to encourage you to eat foods and supplements that are high in iodine, to encourage the thyroid gland to produce hormones. Zinc taken as a supplement will also help boost your hormone balance.

Treat pelvic inflammatory disease

Pelvic inflammatory disease (PID) is a serious set of infections which, if left untreated, could cause infertility. If you have any symptoms of pain in the abdomen, vaginal discharge, or bleeding outside your normal period or ovulatory cycle, combined with painful sex, sickness, or diarrhea, see your physician immediately.

PID may be caused by infection after miscarriage, abortion, or following use of an IUD. It can also be sexually transmitted. Working alongside orthodox health care, complementary approaches will aim to improve the immune system and reduce pain and inflammation, using aromatherapy oils, improved nutrition, and food supplements. Cleansing herbs prescribed by your herbalist, douches to cleanse the affected area, and yogurt to restore bacterial balance are all useful remedies. Improving your absorption of iron, both through foods and supplements, will also aid recovery.

Chapter five

Countdown to conception

Holistic approaches to conception emphasize a working partnership between you and your clinician, building on natural health-care methods. Even if you are told by your clinician to "go away and keep trying," there is much you can do to improve your chances of conceiving.

The countdown to conception on the following pages will boost your fertility and improve your chances of a successful, healthy pregnancy, with a reduced risk of complications.

It is important to inform your clinician about your plans if you are having any kind of medical treatment or are due to undergo surgery. If you have been diagnosed with a condition such as epilepsy, diabetes, or MS, ask if the treatment is likely to affect your fertility and wellbeing, and if there are any side-effects. Find out about complementary treatment options that may reduce side-effects or help you to cut down on your medication levels. If you have any doubts or concerns, don't be afraid to ask more questions or for things to be explained again. It's important that you know the effects any treatment might have on your fertility.

Tests are helpful in pinpointing problems—many of which can then be treated through diet and vitamin and mineral supplements. Fertility tests look for changes in sperm, or unusual signs that may indicate toxic effects. These may be only temporary, and avoiding toxic substances may be enough to improve sperm quality.

One of the most important is the postcoital test, which is used to check the man's sperm levels, the woman's mucus, the strength and activity of sperm in this environment, and the possible presence of antisperm antibodies all at once. The results of this test can rapidly identify typical problems so fertility levels can be restored.

Hair testing, as well as traditional blood tests, is a common and reliable method of identifying heavy metals. Once the cause of any problem has been identified, your nutritional regime can reduce toxic substances by increasing the "turnover rate" in your system and encouraging their elimination. For the same reason, plan a checkup with your dentist as soon as you decide to boost

The healthier you and your partner are before conception, the better chance you have of a trouble-free pregnancy. You will feel happier and more relaxed, knowing that you have done everything possible to insure the wellbeing of your future child.

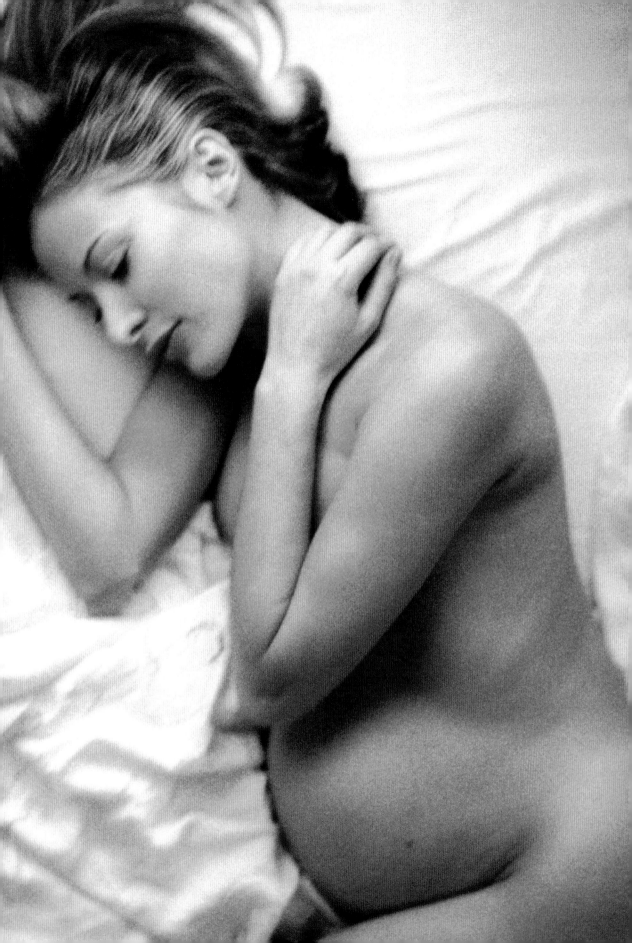

your fertility. Have any necessary treatment before you intend to start trying to conceive, and reduce your mercury levels by improving your diet. Consider having existing amalgam fillings in your teeth replaced.

Assess your environmental hazards at home and at work. Find ways of cutting down your contact with them. Reduce stressful activities, such as rushed meals, long-distance driving, or poor sleep, as far as possible. Try simple massage techniques to improve the quality of the time you spend together.

Use the tables on the following pages as a checklist, adapting them to your situation by highlighting your priorities. This countdown mirrors the nine months of pregnancy, but you can shorten or extend it, depending on your personal circumstances. Don't rush your conception plan: it should be joyful and relaxed. The first few months are packed with action points, but they lessen as the plan continues. You will then develop a routine of good nutrition, exercise, and relaxation—keep it up until you are ready to conceive. You'll be surprised how quickly time flies to that final countdown moment.

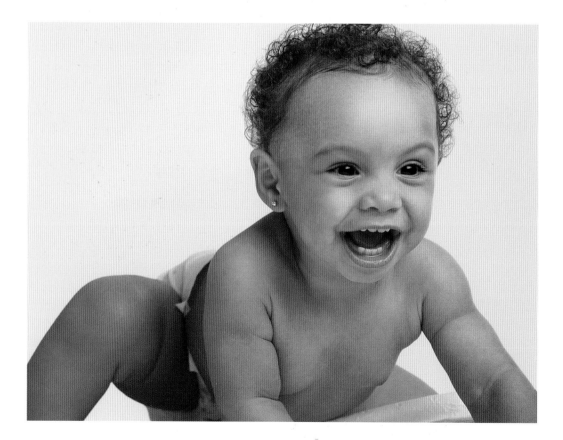

Month nine: ready, steady, go!

Actions: woman

Fertility awareness:

Stop taking contraceptive pill or arrange to have an IUD removed.

Use your agreed alternative method of contraception.

Purchase and familiarize yourself with a basal body temperature thermometer.

Decide whether to purchase and use other technical aids, such as an ovulation predictor, to chart your fertility.

Make nine enlarged photocopies of the chart on page 131.

Begin charting your early morning temperature and note the pattern it takes over the month.

Support your partner in taking steps to improve his sperm count.

➲ Reduce your use of cosmetics and artificially scented products.

Eat plenty of fresh fruit and vegetables to keep your vitamin levels high.

Actions: man

Fertility awareness:

Use your agreed alternative method of contraception.

Find out about detoxifying your body and the dietary and relaxation methods that can improve your sperm count and the strength and motility of your sperm (see Chapters 2 and 3).

Make sure you understand the primary female fertility signs.

Follow your partner's charting and get to know her cycle's signs and symptoms.

Support your partner in learning to use the thermometer for taking her early morning temperature.

Actions: shared

Improve nutrition:

Identify and agree your priorities.

Go through the countdown, checking off completed tasks.

Keep a shared diary of one week's eating habits, including meals not prepared at home and snacks.

Go through the contents of your pantry. Note products made with refined ingredients and additives.

Start cutting down on:

Refined foods containing white flour, sugar, and unnecessary additives.

Your intake of alcohol, artificially sweetened carbonated drinks, tea, coffee, milk substitutes, and sweeteners.

Smoking: use hypnotherapy, acupuncture, or a self-help tape to help you cut down and aim to stop smoking completely by the end of month six.

Steps to health:

Eat fresh, raw, whole, and organic foods whenever possible.

Buy a water filter and use filtered water for all food and drink preparation.

Try healthy "treats" and find some new favorites.

Month eight: A reality check

Actions: woman	**Actions:** man	**Actions:** shared

Health record:

Prepare as full a picture as possible of your family health history; include grandparents if you can.

Note any inherited patterns and potential problems.

Note any food sensitivities, intolerances, or allergies.

Truthfully assess personal smoking and alcohol habits.

Honestly list your drug intake habits, including any "recreational" drugs, self-selected, and prescribed drugs.

Be honest about past and present sexual health and any problems.

Identify and make lists of possible causes of stress at home and at work.

Fertility awareness:

Continue charting your early morning temperature; see if you can identify the day you ovulate.

Start noting your fluid signs and compare them with your temperature changes.

A basal body thermometer helps you record minor fluctuations in temperature.

Health record:

Prepare as full a picture as possible of your family health history; include grandparents if you can.

Note any inherited patterns and potential problems.

Note any food sensitivities, intolerances, or allergies.

Truthfully assess personal smoking and alcohol habits.

Honestly list your drug intake habits, including any "recreational" drugs, self-selected, and prescribed drugs.

Be honest about past and present sexual health and any problems.

Identify and make lists of possible causes of stress at home and at work.

Semen sample tests:

Semen samples are now considered essential for all men undergoing a fertility program and you may need up to three tests.

Make an appointment for your first test.

See your clinician:

Attend all your appointments together.

Take your family health records with you.

Undergo genitourinary examination.

If necessary, have tests to check for possible vitamin and mineral deficiencies and for levels of essential fatty acids and mineral or organic toxins.

Tests may include:

Blood pressure.

Blood, hair, and sweat analysis.

Urine and stool analysis.

See your complementary practitioner:

Take your individual family health records with you.

Explain that you are both working to improve your fertility and reduce your stress levels.

Plan a series of visits to fit in with your countdown to conception timetable.

Your dentist:

Explain your plans and, if fillings are needed, request that they do not contain mercury.

Avoid the use of X-rays. If they are necessary, have them taken now.

Month seven: Step up your action plan

Actions: woman

Identify work hazards:
 VDU screens.
 Chemical exposure.
 Stress factors.
 Other potential occupational
health hazards.

Steps to reduce hazards:
 Talk to your manager,
supervisor, or personnel
officer in confidence about
your plans and concerns.
 Propose and discuss
alternative solutions to
problems—both short-
and long-term.

Fertility awareness:
 Continue charting your
early morning temperature
and fluid signs.
 Compare the temperature
and fluid signs on your chart
and see if you can identify
your fertile phase.
 Begin checking your cervix
position and note it on your
chart.
 Support your partner in
taking sperm count tests and
undergoing therapy.

Actions: man

Identify work hazards:
 VDU screens.
 Chemical exposure.
 Stress factors.
 Other potential occupational
health hazards.

Steps to reduce hazards:
 Talk to your manager,
supervisor, or personnel
officer in confidence about
your plans and concerns.
 Propose and discuss
alternative solutions to
problems—both short-
and long-term.

Fertility awareness:
 If low sperm counts are
identified, therapy will take
place over the next three
months.
 Make an appointment for
your second sperm count test.
 Support your partner in
charting her fertility patterns.

*Regular walks are a safe and
effective form of exercise for
you both.*

Actions: shared

**Follow-up medical
appointment:**
 Review test results.
 Discuss implications
of results.
 Begin course of necessary
vitamin and/or mineral
supplements.
 Start therapies or treatment
for any diagnosed infections.
 Discuss exercise strategies.

**Follow-up complementary
health care sessions:**
 Discuss any reactions
to treatment.
 Review your relaxation
regime.
 Discuss exercise strategies.

Start exercise program:
 Begin light, shared exercise
programs such as yoga, t'ai
chi or other stretching/
relaxing exercise.
 Walking or other gentle
outdoor activity.
 Partner dancing.

**Step up your antismoking
campaign:**
 Create a no-smoking home.
 Warn your friends and
relatives that you are
stopping smoking.
 Ask for support at work.

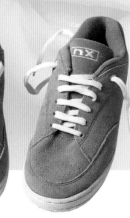

Month six: Bringing it all together

Actions: woman

Fertility awareness:
- Continue charting your early morning temperature, fluid signs, and cervix position.
- Compare the signs recorded on your fertility chart and see if you can identify your fertile phase.
- Begin noting your general body signs.

Essential actions:
- Have rubella immunity test.
- Stop handling cat litter.
- Avoid unpasteurized dairy products.
- Avoid undercooked or raw meats.

Drink plenty of filtered water instead of coffee and tea.

Actions: man

Fertility awareness:
- Continue therapy for low sperm counts, if necessary.
- Make sure you improve your nutrition and take any supplements regularly.
- Keep clothing loose and wear natural materials close to the skin.
- Reduce the number of hours you drive each week.
- Confirm an appointment for your third sperm count test.
- Support your partner in charting her fertility patterns.

Actions: shared

Fertility awareness:
- Review the fertility chart patterns and sperm count results.
- Consider what more you can do to optimize nutrition and improve your wellbeing; for example, cut down further on alcohol intake.

Follow-up actions:
- Make medical appointments if required.
- Continue complementary health-care sessions.
- Continue your exercise regime.

Keep up the good work:
- Make sure as many hazards as possible have been removed from your home and work place.
- Begin your personalized nutrition plan.
- Keep taking vitamin and mineral supplements to boost your fertility.
- Keep filtering your water.
- Stop smoking now!

Month five: Consider your career options

Actions: woman

Fertility awareness:
Continue charting:your early morning temperature, fluid signs, cervix position, and general body signals.

Compare the signs recorded on your fertility chart and be sure you have a regular cycle in which you can identify your fertile phase.

Look at your fertility chart together and discuss what you record.

Actions: man

Fertility awareness:
Complete therapy for low sperm count if necessary.

Keep taking all nutritional supplements to boost fertility levels.

Support your partner in charting her fertility patterns.

Actions: shared

Practical matters:
Check your career options and legal rights on matters such as social security, parental leave, financial benefits, and job-sharing.

Follow-up actions:
Make medical appointments if required.

Continue complementary health-care sessions.

Last chance for dental checkups—make sure treatment is completed before month four.

Continue your exercise and relaxation regime.

Hazards:
Make sure any remaining hazards are removed from your home and work place.

Nutrition:
Continue your nutrition plan.

Keep taking your vitamin and mineral supplements.

Keep filtering your water.

Month four: the holistic program in place

Actions: woman

Finishing touches:
Have your rubella immunization now, if necessary. Do not become pregnant for three months following this.

If possible, cut out the use of VDUs for the three months prior to conception and for the first three months of pregnancy.

Fertility awareness:
Continue charting your early morning temperature, fluid signs, cervix position, and general body signs.

Compare the signs recorded on your fertility chart and be sure you have a regular cycle in which you can identify your fertile phase.

Start counting down three cycles from this month's ovulation.

Visualize your body producing ripe, fertile eggs each month.

Actions: man

Finishing touches:
Keep taking all nutritional supplements to boost fertility levels.

Cut out the use of VDUs for the three months prior to conception.

Continue to support your partner in charting her fertility patterns.

Start counting down ninety days.

Visualize your body developing strong, healthy sperm.

Close your eyes, relax, and visualize your body becoming more and more fertile.

Actions: shared

Make sure that:
Nutrition levels are good and your intake of refined foods and additives is low.

Work place and home hazards are low.

Your exercise regime is reaping benefits.

Your relaxation program is working and you are happy and confident.

You understand your fertile phase and can identify the key signals.

Resolve any outstanding issues:
At home and at work.

With your clinician and complementary practitioner.

With your partner and other members of your family.

With friends.

Remember:
Zero alcohol, smoking, and recreational drugs.

Take only prescribed drugs that your clinician feels are essential.

Month three: the countdown begins

Actions: woman

Reminders:
Trust your chart to tell you the right time to start trying to conceive.
Don't be impatient to conceive if it's not the right time for you.

Actions: man

Reminders:
Is it three months since your final sperm count?
Your sperm will soon be at optimum levels of strength, motility, and number.

Actions: shared

Reminders:
Keep your nutrition and vitality levels high.
Keep a good balance between exercise and relaxation.
Start making extra efforts to be together during your fertile phase.
If you're unsure about lovemaking techniques or want to improve your skills together, buy a book or video tape to boost your confidence.

Month two

Reminders:
Take extra care of yourself and avoid:
Smoky atmospheres and chemicals.
Handling cat litter or strong household cleaners.
Unpasteurized eggs and cheese, raw meat, and fish.

Reminders:
Keep clothing loose.
Wear natural materials close to the skin.
Keep your driving to a minimum.
Stay cool—literally!

Reminders:
Keep using a barrier method of contraception until you are sure you are ready to conceive.
Keep a balance between excitement and stress.

Month one

Reminders:
Is it three months since your rubella immunization?
Use an LH test to check ovulation.
You may not produce an egg every month.
There's still plenty of time.

Reminders:
It only needs one of your millions of sperm to fertilize an egg.
Sperm can live up to five days in a fertile environment.

Reminders:
Give each other a massage.
Book some time off—and stay home alone.
Remember that you don't have to make love unless you truly want to.

Appendix one: Assisted conception

Using the countdown program will boost your fertility and improve your chances of a healthy, natural conception within a few months. It can also improve your chance of successful fertilization if assisted conception is your only possible route to pregnancy. Preexisting medical conditions may dictate a combination approach: use the methods described in this book for achieving your optimum wellbeing, together with one of the assisted conception treatments.

The types of medical conditions that may benefit from assisted conception include some testicular and other cancers affecting men, low or zero sperm count, and immature sperm; spinal injury patients can also benefit. Women who ovulate irregularly or not at all, and those who have blocked fallopian tubes, may also be offered assisted conception treatments. Reversal of earlier vasectomy or fallopian tube interruption is also possible, in certain conditions.

The tables overleaf briefly describe the different treatments involved and raise issues that you may wish to consider before you proceed. Some treatments are very new, and there is little information on their relative success, but advances in medicine mean that fertility services are changing all the time, thanks to new technology and improved laboratory techniques. The techniques, typically, require commitment to regimes lasting several months, and you will be advised about treatments that may carry health risks to you and your future children.

When considering likely success rates, remember that your particular situation is most relevant. However, you will be advised that rates vary between 20 and 30 percent. Be aware that these success figures include only those couples who complete several treatment cycles. Around 10 percent of couples are advised to discontinue treatment, and more than 50 percent choose to stop.

Speak to a qualified counselor who is experienced in fertility issues before you commit yourselves to an assisted conception program. Ask about practical matters, such as diagnostic tests, drug treatments, and the clinical methods used. Take advice about your particular medical condition and which methods may help in your case. Think about how you would feel if your fertility program was not successful. If your treatment regime requires the use of donated sperm or eggs, talk to your partner about how this might affect your relationship and the way you bring up your child.

Use this book to boost your overall health, paying particular attention to your emotional health and relaxation techniques. Check the "five steps to a healthy conception" on page 38, since these will benefit your overall health, regardless of your particular condition. The resources list on pages 138–139 gives additional sources of information, which may be helpful.

How the countdown to conception might help

If either of you is underweight or overweight, suffering from extreme stress, or undergoing a course of tranquilizing drugs, you will usually be advised to address these issues before undergoing assisted conception, since these are typical factors in subfertility. Even a 10 percent weight loss, for example, will improve your chances of conception.

If you smoke—stop now! If you do stop, you have the same chance of a successful conception as nonsmoking couples in assisted reproduction treatments. Similarly, you will be advised to avoid alcohol altogether and cut down on your caffeine intake, particularly in coffee. All of these measures will improve your chances.

For men, taking vitamins C and E can help increase levels of sperm and their quality and motility. Improving your intake of minerals, notably zinc, selenium, magnesium, and potassium, will also help sperm motility and quality. Allow about 90 days for results to show up in sperm tests. For women, taking B-complex vitamins will help counter premenstrual syndrome, and St. John's wort will improve stress or depression.

You might want to book a course of massage or aromatherapy for each of you to help you to stay relaxed during the progress of your treatment. Consider also the potential benefits from complementary health care. For example, acupuncture can improve your sperm count and homeopathy can help to regularize your ovulation cycle.

It is also important to clear up any old infections and candida imbalance. Stick to your treatment regimes, and use vitamin and mineral supplements to increase your vitality. For example, vitamin C will help your body to absorb iron; supplements containing essential fatty acids (EFAs), such as evening primrose oil, will boost your overall fertility levels. Take vitamin and mineral supplements consistently—for at least 30 days—to improve your fertility at cellular level.

Assisted conception: treatment options for men

Treatment name	Description	Potential hazards
Treatment to correct "varicocele" Good for subfertile semen caused by dilated veins.	Caused by impaired drainage into spermatic veins; typically corrected by surgery.	
Artificial insemination by the partner, or AIH Good for men with a low sperm count or weak sperm.	Sperm is injected directly into womb during the fertile phase of a woman's cycle. Success rate is about 30 percent.	Places stress on the man to produce viable sperm; woman must undergo insemination treatment timed to coincide with ovulation.
Artificial insemination by a donor, or AID Typically used for men with very low or zero viable sperm counts, when fertilization is not thought possible.	The same process as above but using donated sperm. The woman receives the donated sperm at the precise time in her fertile cycle.	The "father" responsible for the care of the future child is not the genetic father. Donated sperm may carry genetic faults/infection (despite careful screening).
Fertility drugs Typically used for men with low hormone levels.	Supplements of GnRH, a hormone that promotes growth and function of the gonads, are given.	Success rates are not high.
Intracytoplasmic Injection, (ICSI) Good for men with low sperm count, no motile sperm, or immature sperm.	A single sperm is injected into the ooplasm (the very center of the egg) using a micropipette.	This and the following treatments all involve new technology and have only been carried out on low numbers of people to date.
Subzonal Insemination (SUZI) Good for men with low sperm count, no motile sperm, or immature sperm	Sperm is placed under the zona pellucida (protective coat around the egg) using a micropipette.	
Zona drilling (ZD) Good for men with low sperm count, no motile sperm, or immature sperm	A chemical is applied that dissolves the zona pellucida to create a small hole. Sperm is then placed next to the egg.	

Assisted conception: treatment options for women

Treatment name	Description	Potential hazards
Fertility drugs Given to women who do not ovulate.	Drugs such as "clomiphene citrate" are used to induce ovulation and thus help achieve conception. If the LH surge is low, hormone supplements may be given to improve LH function. Estrogen may be given to enhance sperm penetration by improving the receptivity of cervical mucus.	Possibility of multiple births or toxic side-effects. May exacerbate preexisting pelvic or cervical infection. Concerns about the chances of polycystic ovaries, ovarian hyperstimulation syndrome (OHSS), and ovarian cancer caused by use of fertility drugs. Stimulates production of high numbers of eggs for "harvesting" over a short timespan—possibly using up the egg store.
Tubal surgery Good for blockage of the fallopian tubes.	Removal of adhesions outside the tubes, sometimes by laser treatment.	Less successful for repairing damage to the inner tubal lining.
Gamete intrafallopian transfer, or GIFT	Eggs and sperm are mixed in vitro and then transferred by laparoscope into the woman's fallopian tubes.	Stressful for both partners. The treatment requires both the man and woman to be involved in a precise timetable of activities. If donated eggs are used, the woman is not the genetic mother.
In-vitro fertilization, or IVF Good for blocked or damaged tubes.	Tubes are bypassed by harvesting eggs at time of ovulation. Fertility drugs are used to mature several eggs at once. Eggs are then fertilized outside the womb and then transferred inside by catheter. Eggs may be donated.	If donated eggs are used, the woman is not the genetic mother. Success rate is about 20 to 30 percent.

Appendix two: Charting fertility

Photocopy and enlarge the chart on the opposite page and use it to record your cycle changes and to help you recognize your fertile time. You will need a basal body thermometer, available from pharmacies, for taking your temperature. This records very slight variations, and it may take you a little while to get used to reading it. Take your temperature, placing the thermometer in your mouth for five minutes, then jot down the reading on your chart. Do this first thing in the morning when you wake, before getting up or having a hot drink.

Additional notes for your chart

Try to record your basal body temperature as accurately as possible, using the points on the chart where the lines meet. Each degree is divided into 10 points, so you should get a clear reading. Add notes about your background body signals, levels of sexual desire, vaginal fluids, and cervical position to your chart to give a complete fertility picture. The following are suggestions as to how you might develop your chart. Don't worry if you don't experience all these signals. They are simply examples of the type of feelings and signs some women have.

Background body signals:
Use a pattern, such as * or #, to indicate signals, followed by initials to specify the signal.
For example:
A&P: aches and pains
SP: spotting
T: tingling
BP: bowel pressure

Peaks and dips of hormonal levels tend to coincide with sexual desire. Use arrows to show record your sexual feelings:
↗ Increased energy and sexual desire
↘ Tiredness or irritability, decrease in energy

Vaginal fluids:
Use key words such as "dry," "sticky," or "acid" to indicate the infertile days in your cycle or "damp," "clear,"or "abundant" to describe your fertile phase.

Cervix changes:
Use initials to describe the position of the cervix:
L: Lower—infertile
H: Higher—fertile phase
Your physician can show you how to check your cervical position.

You can also chart your LH surge (see pages 76–77), using a home-testing kit. Follow the instructions carefully and note the results in the background-signals box on the relevant day or days. A pattern will emerge, and you should be able to identify your most fertile phase after about three months of keeping a chart.

Once you have created an overall picture of your monthly cycle, you may wish to highlight your fertile phase—probably two to five days in the middle of your cycle. Use a color—such as green—to indicate the outer days, and a brighter shade of the color to pinpoint the day on which you ovulate.

Countdown to conception

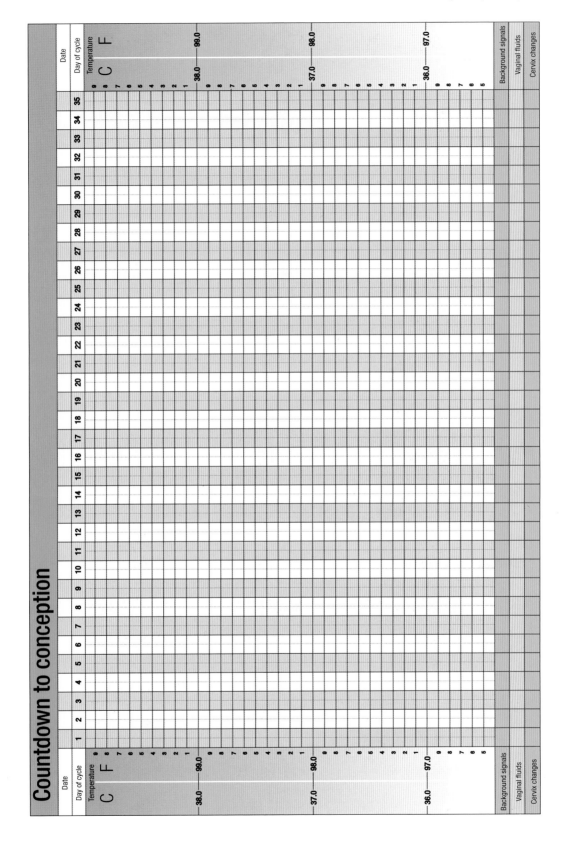

Keeping a lifestyle diary

When you begin your countdown-to-conception plan, start keeping a lifestyle diary. Get into the habit of writing down everything you eat and drink—including those items you know you shouldn't have had! Keep a record of how much exercise you take, your sleep patterns, even how you feel. Over the weeks you will become aware of emerging patterns, such as whether you always get a headache after eating a particular item or need more sleep at certain times of the month. Your diary will help you avoid these "bad" triggers and encourage better habits. Use your diary to help you remember targeted lifestyle changes, too, such as drinking more filtered water or taking your food supplements regularly.

Monday
Massage appointments for us both—4 and 4.30. Walked home (30 minutes). Breakfast: two slices of toast and honey, apple, Lunch: cheese and tomato sandwich. Dinner: pasta with chicken and mushrooms. Drinks: 2 coffee, 2 tea, 1 glass of water. Snacks: 1 chocolate bar, 2 cookies.

Tuesday
Test results—low sperm count. Didn't manage any exercise. Felt very tired and stressed—period due soon? Breakfast: toast and jelly. Lunch: pasta and tomato sauce. Dinner: baked potato and salad. Drinks: 1 coffee, 2 herbal tea, 2 glasses water. Snacks: 1 apple, 1 banana.

Wednesday
Spoke to boss about VDUs. Put no smoking signs around desk. Went swimming. Felt tired but relaxed afterward. Breakfast: toast, orange juice. Lunch: pizza and salad. Dinner: chicken and rice, Drinks: 2 tea, 1 coffee, 3 glasses water, Snacks: grapes.

Thursday
Arrange supply of organic milk. Breakfast: granola with organic fruit. Lunch: toasted sandwich. Dinner: take-out chili. Drinks: 1 juice, 2 water, 1 coffee, 1 tea Snacks: candy bar, 7.30p.m. started dance class—good exercise and fun.

Friday
Indigestion—chili? Very tired—period due, No exercise, Meat-free day: Breakfast: grape-fruit, granola, Lunch: cottage cheese and salad, Dinner: vegetable lasagne, strawberries. Drinks: 1 herbal tea, 1 coffee (decaf) 3 glasses water, 1 juice, Snack: cookie (must stop these).

Saturday
Period started . Began fertility chart. Slight headache in morning. Change water filter, Exercise: gardening. Breakfast: granola, toast, juice, Lunch: BLT sandwich, Dinner: seafood restaurant, Drinks: 1 tea, 2 coffee (decaf), 2 water, 1 juice, 1 white wine.

Sunday
Dinner with parents-in-law—ask about J's childhood illnesses. Walk in park. Breakfast: toast, fruit. Lunch: omelet and salad. Dinner: vegetable soup, chicken, potatoes, broccoli, ice cream. Drinks: 3 coffee, 4 water, 1 herbal tea. Slept badly—late dinner?

Reminders
Book time off to paint bedroom? Put in request for water machine in office. Buy toxin-absorbing plants for desk. Clear out chemicals from workshop. Next week aim to cut down on coffee, tea, and cookies, eat more fruit, and drink more water.

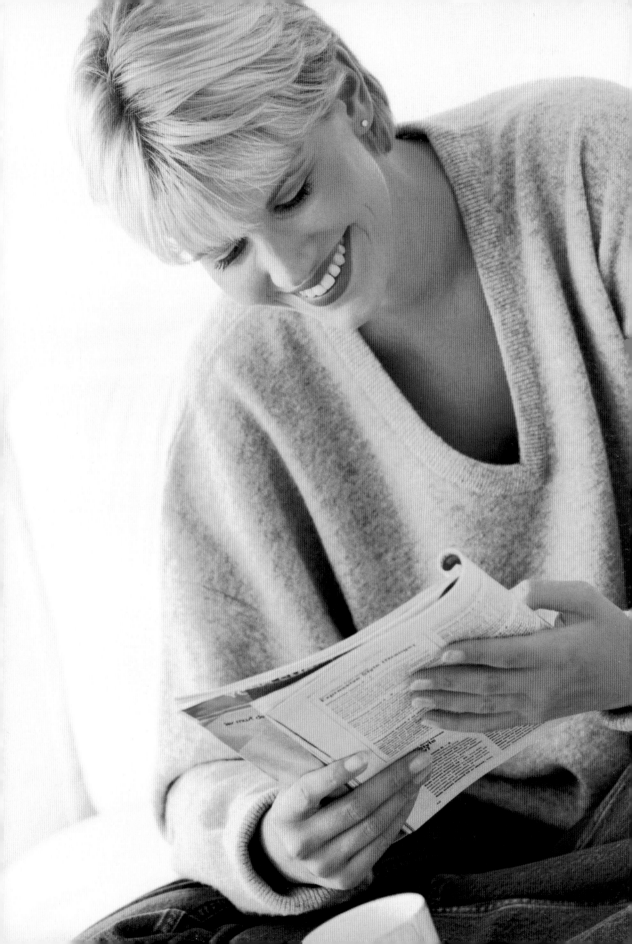

Bibliography

FORESIGHT INFORMATION BOOKLETS
Preparing for Pregnancy
The Health Professionals' Guide to Preconception Care,
Dr. M. Glenville.
Chapter from *Vitamins in Endocrine Metabolism,*
Jenning S., (first published by William Heinemann,
Medical Press, 1972.)
The following booklets are all by T. Tuormaa:
*The Adverse Effects of Manganese Deficiency on
Reproduction*
The Adverse Effects of Alcohol on Reproduction
The Adverse Effects of Tobacco Smoking on Reproduction
The Adverse Effects of Food Additives on Health
The Adverse Effects of Genito-Urinary Infections
The Adverse Effects of Zinc Deficiency
*The Adverse Effects of Agro-chemicals on Reproduction
and Health*
The Adverse Effects of Lead

BASIC REFERENCES
Essential Reproduction , Martin H. Johnson, Barry J.
Everitt, Blackwell Science Ltd., 1995.
Stedman's Concise Medical & Allied Health Dictionary,
Ed. John H. Dirckx, MD, Williams & Wilkins,
1997.

FURTHER READING
Acupressure for Common Ailments, Chris Jarmey &
John Tindall, Simon & Schuster, 1991.
Aromatherapy for Common Ailments, Shirley Price,
Simon & Schuster, 1991.
The Book of Ayurveda: a guide to personal wellbeing,
Judith H. Morrison, Simon & Schuster, 1995.
Chinese System of Food Cures, Henry C. Lu, Sterling
Publishing, 1986.
The Complete Woman's Herbal, Anne McIntyre,
Henry Holt, 1994.
Diabetes, R. Tattersall, Churchill Livingstone, 1986.
The Doctor's Book of Home Remedies for Women, Ed.
Sharon Faelten, Rodale Press, 1997.
Encyclopaedia of Complementary Medicine by Anne
Woodham & Dr. David Peters, Dorling Kindersley,
1997.
Epilepsy, P. Hazeldine, Thorsons, 1986.
The Family Guide to Reflexology, Ann Gillanders,
Little, Brown, 1998.

*Fertility: fertility awareness and natural family
planning,* Dr. E. Clubb & J. Knight, David &
Charles, 1996.
Healing Foods for Common Ailments, Dr. Penny
Stanway, Key Porter, 1995.
Herbs for Common Ailments, Anne McIntyre, Simon
& Schuster, 1992.
Homeopathy for Common Ailments, Robin Hayfield,
Frog Ltd., 1993.
The Joy of Reflexology, Ann Gillanders, Little, Brown,
1995.
The Manual of Natural Family Planning, Dr. A.M.
Flynn & M. Brooks, Thorsons, 1996.
Massage for Common Ailments, Sara Thomas, Barnes
and Noble, 1989.
Natural Fertility Awareness, J. & L. Davidson, The
C.W. Daniel Company Ltd., 1994.
New Choices in Natural Healing, Ed. Bill Gottlieb,
Rodale Press, 1995.
The New Natural House Book, David Pearson, Simon
& Schuster, 1998.
*New Natural Pregnancy: practical wellbeing from
conception to birth,* Janet Balaskas, Interlink, 1999.
Our Toxic World: who is looking after our kids?, Harold
E. Buttram, MD, Richard Piccola, MHA,
Foresight/America Foundation for Preconception
Care, 1996.
The Reflexology Handbook: a complete guide, L.
Norman and T. Cowan, Judy Piatkus Ltd., 1988.
Taking Charge of Your Fertility, Toni Weschler, MPH,
HarperCollins, 1995.
Understanding Endometriosis, C. Hawkridge,
MacDonald Optima, 1989
Women's Guide to Homeopathy, Andrew Lockie and
Nicola Geddes, Hamish Hamilton, 1993.
Yoga for Common Ailments, Dr. Nagendra, Dr.
Nagarathna, Dr. Robin Monro, Simon & Schuster,
1990.

PAMPHLETS AND BROCHURES
A Window on Fertility and Conception, Unipath Ltd.,
Priory Business Park, Bedford MK44 3UP, UK (011
44 1234 835000)
*From Small Beginnings…First Steps to Starting a
Family,* Unipath Limited, Priory Business Park,
Bedford MK44 3UP, UK (011 44 1234 835000)

Fertility (ovulation or basal) Thermometer, G.H. Zeal Ltd., 8 Deer Park Road, London SW19 3UU, UK (011 44 20 8542 2283)

How to Remove Old Lead Paint Safely, British Coating Federation, James House, Bridge Street, Leatherhead, Surrey KT22 7EP, UK (011 44 1372 360660)

MS Matters, MS Society, 25 Effie Road, London SW6 1EE, UK (011 44 20 7610 7171). Helpline 011 44 20 7371 8000; Info@mssociety.org.uk

Official Journal of the European Commission:
Parental Leave Directive: 96/34. Journal No. L145/96
Extending Parental Leave to UK: 97/75.Journal No. L10/98
Maternity Leave: 92/85.Journal No. L348/92

Information on Clomiphene:
www.healthnet.ivi.com/pharm/html/002151.htm?Clomid

Abstracts from MEDLINE
www.healthgate.com/medline/search-medline.shtml
General enquiries: info@healthgate.com
Telephone: 781-685–4000

1. Laparoscopic surgery in infertile women with minimal or mild endometriosis. Marcoux-S; Maheus-R; Berube-S., *N.Engl.J.Med.* 1997 Jul.

2. Testicular cancer and spermatogenesis. Botchan-A; Hauser-R; Yogev-L; Gamzu-R; Paz-G; Lessing-JB; Yavetz-H. *Hum. Reprod.,* 1997 Apr.

3. Evidence for regional differences of semen quality among fertile French men. Auger-J; Jouannet-P; *Hum. Reprod.* 1997 Apr.

4. Effects of psychological stress on human semen quality. Fenster-L; Katz-DF; Wyrobek-AJ; Pieper-C; Rempel-DM; Oman-D; Swan-SH. *J.Androl.* 1997, Mar–Apr.

5. Predicting optimal cervical mucus for infertility diagnosis. Oei-SG; Helmerhorst-FM; Bloemenkamp-KW; Dersjant-Roorda-M; Kerse-MJ. *Eur.J.Obstet.Gynecol.Reprod.Biol.,* 1997 May.

6. Assessment of reproductive disorders and birth defects in communities near hazardous chemical sites. III. Guidelines for field studies of male reproductive disorders. Wyrobek-AJ; Schrader-SM; Perreault-SD; Fenster-L; Huszar-G; Katz-DF; Osorio-AM; Sublet-V;Evenson-D. *Reprod.Toxicol.* 1997, Mar–Jun.

7. Sexuality and fertility in long-term survivors of testicular cancer. Arai-Y; Kawakita-M; Okada-Y; Yoshida-O; *J.Clin.Oncol.* 1997 Apr.

8. Physical complaints and emotional stress related to routine diagnostic procedures of the fertility investigation. Eimers-JM; Omtzigt-AM; Vogelzang-ET; van-Ommen-R; Habbema-JD; te-Velder-ER. *J. Psychosom.Obstet.Gynaecol.* 1997 Mar.

9. Environmental factors which impair male fertility. Indulski-JA; Sitarek-K; *Med.Pr.* 1977.

10. The effect of human papillomavirus infection on sperm cell motility. Lai-YM; Lee-JF; Huang-HY; Soong-YK; Yang-FP; Pao-CC; *Fertil.Steril.* 1997 Jun.

11. Therapy of male subfertility. Schill-WB; Kohn-FM; *Wien.Med. Wochenschr.* 1997.

12. Role of hypo-osmotic sperm swelling test in assisted reproduction. Datta-S; Giri-A; Datta-AK. *J.Indian Med. Assoc.* 1996 Dec.

13. Evaluation of luteal phase in normal and infertile women. John-M; Rameshkumar-K; Lillian-DA. *Indian J. Pathol. Microbiol.* 1997 Jan.

14. Occupational exposures and risk of female infertility. Smith-EM; Hammonds-Ehlers-M; Clark-MK; Kirchner-HL; Furotes-L. *J.Occup.Environ. Med.* 1997 Feb.

15. Occupational reproductive hazards. Paul-M. *Lancet* 1997 May.

16. Anaerobes in ejaculates of subfertile men. Eggert-Kruse-W; Rohr-G; Strock-W; Pohl-S; Schwalback-B; Runnebaum-B; *Hum.Reprod.Update.* 1995 Sep.

17. Human semen analysis; Comharie-F; Vermeulen-L. *Hum.Reprod.Update.* 1995 Jul.

18. Motherhood, motherliness, and psychogenic infertility. Allison-GH. *Psychoanal-Q* 1997 Jan.

19. Electroejaculation and assisted reproductive techniques in the patients with spinal cord injury. Yamamoto-M; Yamada-K; Hirata-N; Hirayama-A; Kashiwai-H; Momse-H; Suemori-T; Shiomi-T; Hirao-Y; Okajima-E. *Nippon-Hinyokika.*

Gakkai.Zasshi. 1997 Mar.

20. Sperm quality in Hodgkin's disease versus non-Hodgkin's lymphoma. Botchan-A; Hauser-R; Gamzu-R; Yogev-L; Lessing-JB; Paz-G; Yavetz-H. *Hum. Reprod.* 1997 Jan.

21. Characterization of human sperm antigens reacting with antisperm antibodies from autologous sera and seminal plasma: comparison among infertile subpopulations. Paradisi-R; Bellavia-E; Pession-AL; Venturoli-S; Bach-V; Flamigni-C. *Int.J.Androl.* 1996 Dec.

22. Smoking and male reproduction: a review. Vine-MF. *Int.J.Androl.* 1996 Dec.

23. How should a man with testicular cancer be counselled and what information is available to him? Reiker-PP. SEmin.*Urol. Oncol.* 1996 Feb.

24. Spontaneous pregnancy in couples waiting for artificial insemination donor because of severe male infertility. Matorras-R; Diez-J; Corcostegui-B; Gutierrez-de-Teran-G; Garcia-JM; Pijoan-JI; Rodriguez-Escudero-FJ. *Eur.J.Obstet.Gynecol. Reprod. Biol.* 1996 Dec.

25. Varicocelectromy. Mellinger-BC. *Tech.Urol.* 1995 Winter.

26. Semen analysis of military personnel associated with military duty assignments. Weyandt-TB; Schrader-SM; Turner-TW; Simon-SD. *Reprod.Toxicol.* 1996 Nov-Dec.

27. Couples and reproductive health: a review of couple studies. Becker-S. *Stud.Fam.Plann.* 1996 Nov-Dec.

28. Effects of Panax Ginseng C.A. Meyer saponins on male fertility. Salvati-G; Genovesi-G; Marcellini-L; Paolini-P; De-Nuccio-I; Pepe-M; Re-M. *Panminerva Med.* 1996 Dec.

29. Intracytoplasmic injection with late spermatids: a successful procedure in achieving childbirth for couples in which the male partner suffers from azoospermia due to deficient spermatogenesis. Araki-Y; Motoyama-M; Yoshida-A; Kim-SY; Sung-H; Araki-S. *Fertil.Steril.* 1997 Mar.

30. Evaluation of Infertility. Campana-A; de-Agostini-A; Bischof-P; Tawfik-E; Mastrorilli-A; *Hum.Reprod.Update.* 1995 Nov.

31. Contribution of andrological factors to sterility. Krause-W. *Andrologia* 1996.

32. Andrologic diagnosis today. Haidl-G.

Fortschr.Med. 1996 Dec.

33. Ovulation induction and ovarian malignancy. Beltsos-AN; Odem-RR. *Semin.Reprod. Endocrinol.* 1996 Nov.

34. Reproductive toxicity of ovulation induction. Tucker-KE. *Semin. Reprod. Endocrinol.* 1996 Nov.

35. Cryptorchidism and fertility: evaluation in adult age. D'Agostino-S;Zen-F; Ioverno-E; Pesce-C; Belloli-G. *Pediatr.Med.Chir.* 1996 Sep–Oct.

36. Varicocele: epidemiologic study and indications for its treatment. D'Agostino-S; Musi-L; Colombo-B; Belloli-G. *Pediatr.Med.Chir.* 1996 Sep–Oct.

37. Fallopian tube anastomosis procedures to restore fertility. Haspel-Siegel-AS. *AORN-J.* 1997 Jan.

38. Microsurgery and changes in the testicular and epididymal production of spermatozoa. Sica-GS; Di-Lorenzo-N; Sileri-P; Gaspari-AL. *Ann.Ital.Chir.* 1996 Sep–Oct.

39. The influence of semen analysis parameters on the fertility potential of infertile couples. Ayala-C; Steinberger-E; Smith-DP. *J.Androl.* 1996 Nov–Dec.

40. The intracytoplasmic spermatozoa injection – the way out of the "male fertility crisis"?. Michelmann-HW. *Dtsch. Tierarztl. Wochenschr.* 1996 Oct.

41. Effects of prolonged autovehicle driving on male reproduction function: a study among taxi drivers. Figa-Talamanca-I; Cini-C; Varricchio-GC; Dondero-F; Gandini-L; Lenzi-A; Lombardo-F; Angelucci-L; Di-Grezia-R; Patacchioli-FR. *Am.J.Ind.Med.* 1996 Dec.

42. Evaluation of internal alpha-particle radiation exposure and subsequent fertility among a cohort of women formerly employed in the radium dial industry. Schieve-LA; Davis-F; Roeske-J; Handler-A; Freels-S; Stinchcomb-T; Keane-A; *Radiat.Res.* 1997 Feb.

43. Pregnancy in women undergoing a kidney transplant. Our experience and a review of the literature. Tommasi-GV; Casolino-V; Fontana-I; Beatini-M; Semino-A; Manolitsi-O; Dondero-F; Valente-U. *Minerva-Ginecol.* 1996 Dec.

44. Seminal volume and total sperm number trends in men attending subfertility clinics in the greater Athens area during the period 1977–1993. Adamopoulos-DA; Pappa-A; Nicopoulou-S; Andreou-E; Karamertzanis-M; Michopoulos-J;

Deligianni-V; Simou-M. *Hum.Reprod.* 1996 Sep.

45. The relationship of the postcoital test and semen characteristics to pregnancy rates in 200 presumed fertile couples. Beltsos-AN; Fisher-S; Uhler-ML; Clegg-ED; Zinaman-M; *Int.J. Fertil. Menopausal. Stud.* 1996 Jul–Aug.

46. Vaginal lubricants for the infertile couple: effect on sperm activity. Kutteh-WH;Chao-CH; Ritter-JO; Byrd-W; *Int.J.Fertil.Menopausal Stud.* 1996 Jul–Aug.

47. Adult-onset idiopathic hypogonadotropic hypogonadism – a treatable form of male infertility. Nachtigall-LB: Boepple-PA; Pralong-FP; Crowley-WF Jr. *N.Engl.J.Med.* 1997 Feb.

48. Unfulfilled desire for children in the man: coping and pain. Results of a psychosomatic-andrologic cooperative study. Schilling-S; Kuchenhoff-J; Konnecke-R; Tilgen-W. *Hautarzt.* 1996 Sep.

49. The effects of temperature on human fertility. Lam-DA; Miron-JA; *Demography.* 1996 Aug.

50. Shift work, nitrous oxide exposure and subfertility among Swedish midwives. Ahlborg-G Jr; Axelsson-G; Bodin-L. *Int.J. Epidemiol.* 1996 Aug.

51. The aetiology and management of erectile, ejaculatory, and fertility problems in men with diabetes mellitus. Dunsmuir-WD; Holmes-Sa. *Diabet.Med.* 1996 Aug.

52. Role of oxidative stress and antioxidants in male infertility. Sikka-SC; Rajasekaran-M; Hellstrom-WJ. *J.Androl.* 1995.

53. Infertility and coeliac disease. Collin-P; Vilska-S; Heinonen-PK; Hallstrom-O; Pikkarainen-P. *Gut.* 1996 Sep.

54. Selenium–vitamin E supplementation in infertile men. Effects on semen parameters and micronutrient levels and distribution. Vezina-D; Mauffette-F; Roberts-KD; Bleau-G. *Biol.Trace.Elem.Res.* 1996 Summer.

55. Maternal age effect on early human embryonic development and blastocyst formation. Janny-L; Menezo-YJ. *Mol.Reprod.Dev.* 1996 Sep.

56. Control of fertility by metabolic cues. Wade-GN; Schneider-JE; Li-HY. *Am.J.Physiol.* 1996 Jan.

57. Infertility and subfertility in Norwegian women aged 40–42. Prevalence and factors. Sundby-J; Schei-B. *Acta.Obstet.Gynecol.Scand.* 1996 Oct.

58. Mercury in urine and ejaculate in husbands of barren couples. Hanf-V; Forstmann-A; Costea-JE; Schieferstein-G; Fischer-I; Schweinsberg-F. *Toxicol. Lett.* 1996 Nov.

59. Male fertility following spinal cord injury: facts and fiction. Brackett-NL; Nash-MS; Lynne-CM. *Phys.Ther.* 1996 Nov.

60. The effects of smoking on ovarian function and fertility during assisted reproduction cycles. Van-Voorhis-BJ; Dawson-JD; Stovall-DW; Sparks-AE; Syrop-CH. *Obstet-Gynecol.* 1996 Nov.

61. Cigarette smoking may affect meiotic maturation of human oocytes. Zenzes-MT; Wang-P; Casper-RF. *Hum.Reprod.* 1995 Dec.

62. The effect of smoking and varicocele on human sperm acrosin activity and acrosome reaction. El-Mulla-KF; Kohn-FM; El-Beheiry-AH; Schill-WB. *Hum.Reprod.* 1995 Dec.

63. Varicocele: indications for treatment. Comhaire-F; Zalata-A; Schoonjans-F. Int.J.Androl. 1995 Dec.

64. Immunological aspects of subfertility. Eggert-Krse-W; Rohr-G; Bockem-Hellwig-S; Huber-K; Christmann-Edoga-M; Runnebaum-B. *Int.J.Androl.* 1995 Dec.

65. Does cigarette smoking impair natural or assisted fucundity? Hughes-EG; Brennan-BG. *Fertil.Steril.* 1996 Nov.

66. The new antiepileptic drugs and women: efficacy, reproductive health, pregnancy and fetal outcome. Morrell-MJ. *Epilepsia.* 1996.

67. A group program for obese, infertile women: weight loss and improved psychological health. Galletly-C; Clark-A; Tomlinson-L; Blaney-F. *J.Psychosom.Obstet.Gynaecol.* 1996 Jun.

68. Psychological characteristics of infertile patients: discriminating etiological factors from reactive changes. Stoleru-S; Teglas-JP; Spira-A; Magnin-F; Fermanian-J. *J.Psychosom.Obstet.Gynaecol.* 1996 Jun.

Resources

WOMEN'S HEALTH/WOMEN'S ISSUES WEBSITES

www.women.com

www.mediconsult.com

www.healthgate.com

www.womenshealth.com

www.ivillage.com

WORKPLACE ISSUES

U.S. Equal Employment Opportunity Commission
1801 L Street, N.W.
Washington, D.C. 20507
(202) 663-4900
www.eeoc.gov

FERTILITY AND PRECONCEPTIONAL PLANNING

Foresight/America
10 East Randolph Street
New Hope, PA 18938

Planned Parenthood Federation of America
810 Seventh Avenue
New York, NY 10019
(212) 541-7800
www.plannedparenthood.com
email: communications@ppfa.com

RESOLVE, The National Infertility Association
1310 Broadway
Somerville, MA 02144
(617) 623-0744
www.resolve.org
email: resolveinc@aol.com

International Council on Infertility Information
Dissemination
P.O. Box 6836
Arlington, VA 22206
(703) 379-9178
www.inciid.org
email:INCIIDinfo@inciid.org

Unipath, Ltd.
Priory Business Park
Bedford, MK44 3UP
UK
(011) 44 1234 835000
US Website: www.unipath.com

INFORMATION ABOUT PREEXISTING CONDITIONS

Multiple Sclerosis
The National Multiple Sclerosis Society
733 Third Avenue
New York, NY 10017
1-800-344-4867
www.nmss.org
email: info@nmss.org

Epilepsy
The Epilepsy Foundation
4351 Garden City Drive
Landover, MD 20785
1-800-EFA-1000
www.efa.org
email: info@efa.org

Kidney Disease
National Kidney Foundation
30 East 33rd Street, Suite 1100
New York, NY 10016
1-800-622-9010
www.kidney.org
email: info@kidney.org

HOLISTIC HEALTH CARE
National Center for Complementary and
Alternative Medicine
NCCAM Clearinghouse
P.O. Box 8218
Silver Spring, MD 20907-8218
1-888-644-6226
www.nccam.nig.gov

National Institute of Ayurvedic Medicine
584 Milltown Road
Brewster, NY 10509
(914) 278-8700
www.niam.com

American Yoga Association
P.O. Box 19986
Sarasota, FL 34276
(941) 927-4977

Flower Essence Society
P.O. Box 459
Nevada City, CA 95959
1-800-736-9222
email: mail@flowersociety.org
www.flowersociety.org

North American Society of Homeopaths (NASH)
1122 East Pike Street, Suite 1122
Seattle, WA 98122
(541) 345-9815
www.homeopathy.org

American Association of Naturopathic Physicians
601 Valley Street, Suite 105
Seattle, WA 98109
(206) 298-0126
www.naturopathic.org

American Massage Therapy Association
820 Davis Street, Suite 100
Evanston, IL 60201-4444
(847) 864-0123
www.amtamassage.org

Index

Photo Credits

DigitalVision: 1, 2, 3, 6, 7, 11, 19, 24, 27, 39, 43, 66, 67, 118, 132

Gus Filgate: 50/51, 58/59, 100/101, 106/107

Paul Forrester: 12, 31,119-124, 132

Robert Harding: 37, 103

Ray Moller: 102

Photodisc: 5, 92, 93,

Science Photo Library
Scott Camzine/CDC: 35
K.H. Kjeldsen: 47
Prof. P. Mottra/University "La Sapienza" Rome: 78
Dr. Tony Brain: 89
CNRI: 91
Tim Malyon & Paul Biddle: 105

Tony Stone Images: 22, 69, 97, 105, 116

Artwork

Michael Woods 72–77

Author's Acknowledgments

During the two years that this book has been researched and written, many people have offered information and support, for which I am profoundly grateful. Some have called me with case studies but asked for their names to be changed. This is my opportunity to say thank you for having the courage to talk about your lives.

Others, such as Bill Feeney, Dr. Andy Lockie, Andrew Ward, and Charles Buck, have provided practical information and resources for readers. Yet others have inspired and supported my work, probably without realizing it! Here I would include Heather Campbell, who helped me understand the importance of relaxation and stress management.

Thanks too to Eleanor Lines of Gaia Books, who encouraged me to write this book all that time ago and supported me through some critical moments! Also to the Gaia team who have taken a lot of trouble to present the information in an attractive and accessible way. Dr. Damien Downing and Dr. Helen Dziemidko deserve special commendation for checking the text and making constructive suggestions.

Without Belinda Barnes, of Foresight, this book could not have been written and her dedication to families everywhere deserves wide praise. In the United States, Hal Buttram is doing a tremendous amount to raise awareness of the importance of preconceptional care.

Finally, I would like to thank my family and particularly my partner Bob, who by seeing his name in print can rest assured that this project is finally complete!